New Directions in Nursing Education

Editor

MARY ELLEN SMITH GLASGOW

NURSING CLINICS
OF NORTH AMERICA

www.nursing.theclinics.com

Consulting Editor
SUZANNE S. PREVOST

December 2012 • Volume 47 • Number 4

ELSEVIER

1600 John F. Kennedy Blvd., Suite 1800 • Philadelphia, PA 19103-2899

http://www.theclinics.com

NURSING CLINICS OF NORTH AMERICA Volume 47, Number 4
December 2012 ISSN 0029-6465, ISBN-13: 978-1-4557-4908-9

Editor: Katie Hartner
Developmental Editor: Stephanie Carter

Nursing Clinics of North America (ISSN 0029-6465) is published quarterly by Elsevier Inc., 360 Park Avenue South, New York, NY 10010-1710. Months of issue are March, June, September, and December. Periodicals postage paid at New York, NY and additional mailing offices. Subscription price per year is, $144.00 (US individuals), $360.00 (US institutions), $260.00 (international individuals), $440.00 (international institutions), $210.00 (Canadian individuals), $440.00 (Canadian institutions), $79.00 (US students), and $129.00 (international students). To receive student/resident rate, orders must be accompanied by name of affiliated institution, date of term, and the signature of program/residency coordinator on institution letterhead. Orders will be billed at individual rate until proof of status is received. Foreign air speed delivery is included in all *Clinics* subscription prices. All prices are subject to change without notice. **POSTMASTER:** Send address changes to *Nursing Clinics,* Elsevier Health Sciences Division, Subscription Customer Service, 3251 Riverport Lane, Maryland Heights, MO 63043. **Customer Service: Telephone: 1-800-654-2452** (U.S. and Canada); **1-314-447-8871 (outside U.S. and Canada). Fax: 1-314-447-8029. E-mail: journalscustomerservice-usa@elsevier.com** (for print support) and **journalsonlinesupport-usa@elsevier.com** (for online support).

Nursing Clinics of North America is covered in *EMBASE/Excerpta Medica, MEDLINE/PubMed (Index Medicus), Social Sciences Citation Index, Current Contents, ASCA, Cumulative Index to Nursing, RNdex Top 100,* and Allied Health Literature and International Nursing Index (INI).

Printed in the United States of America.

RT
I
N77
v.47
no.4

Contributors

CONSULTING EDITOR

SUZANNE S. PREVOST, PhD, RN, COI
Associate Dean, Practice and Community Engagement, University of Kentucky, Lexington, Kentucky

GUEST EDITOR

MARY ELLEN SMITH GLASGOW, PhD, RN, ACNS-BC
Dean and Professor, Duquesne University, School of Nursing, Pittsburgh, Pennsylvania

AUTHORS

SANDRA BELLINI, DNP, APRN, NNP-BC, CNE
Associate Clinical Professor and Coordinator, DNP and NNP Programs, School of Nursing, University of Connecticut, Storrs, Connecticut

ANAND BHATTACHARYA, MHS
Independent Statistical Consultant, Secane, Pennsylvania

THERESA CARROLL, PhD
Assistant Dean, Office of Student and Academic Affairs, School of Nursing, University of Virginia, Charlottesville, Virginia

STEPHEN J. CAVANAGH, PhD, MPA, RN, FRSPH, FinstLM
Dean and Professor, School of Nursing, University of Massachusetts Amherst, Amherst, Massachusetts

FRANCES H. CORNELIUS, PhD, RN-BC, CNE
Clinical Associate Professor, Department of Armed Nursing Roles, College of Nursing & Health Professions, Drexel University, Philadelphia, Pennsylvania

REGINA M. CUSSON, PhD, NNP-BC, APRN, FAAN
Professor and Interim Dean, School of Nursing, University of Connecticut, Storrs, Connecticut

H. MICHAEL DREHER, PhD, RN, FAAN
Associate Professor, Department of Armed Nursing Roles, College of Nursing & Health Professions, Drexel University, Philadelphia, Pennsylvania

LYNNE M. DUNPHY, APRN, FNP-BC, PhD
Center Director, Rhode Island Center for Nursing Excellence (RICNE), Routhier Chair of Practice and Professor, College of Nursing, University of Rhode Island, Kingston, Rhode Island

DANA FARABAUGH, MD
Assistant Professor, Department of Obstetrics and Gynecology, Drexel University College of Medicine, Philadelphia, Pennsylvania

DORRIE K. FONTAINE, RN, PhD, FAAN
Dean and Sadie Heath Cabaniss Professor of Nursing, School of Nursing, University of Virginia, Charlottesville, Virginia

MARCIA R. GARDNER, PhD, RN, CPNP, CPN
Associate Professor, Department of Family Nursing, College of Nursing, Seton Hall University, South Orange, New Jersey

ELLEN GIARELLI, EdD, MA, BSN, BS
Associate Professor, College of Nursing and Health Professions, Drexel University, Philadelphia, Pennsylvania

SHARON GRISWOLD-THEODORSON, MD, MPH
Associate Professor, Simulation Center Director, Department of Emergency Medicine, Drexel University College of Medicine, Philadelphia, Pennsylvania

ELYTA H. KOH, MBA
Associate Dean for Administration, School of Nursing, University of Virginia, Charlottesville, Virginia

ROSALIE O. MAINOUS, PhD, APRN, NNP-BC
Dean and Professor, Miami Valley College of Nursing and Health, Wright State University, Dayton, Ohio

PAULA McCAULEY, DNP, APRN, ACNP-BC, CNE
Associate Clinical Professor and Interim Associate Dean, School of Nursing, University of Connecticut, Storrs, Connecticut

FAYE MELOY, PhD, MSN, MBA, RN
Assistant Dean, Pre-licensure BSN Programs, Chair, BSN Co-op Department, College of Nursing and Health Professions, Drexel University, Philadelphia, Pennsylvania

KYMBERLEE MONTGOMERY, DrNP, APRN, WHNP-BC, CNE
Assistant Clinical Professor, Chair, Nurse Practitioner Programs, Drexel University College of Nursing and Health Professions, Drexel University College of Medicine, Philadelphia, Pennsylvania

OWEN MONTGOMERY, MD, FACOG
Associate Professor, Chairman, Department of Obstetrics and Gynecology, Drexel University College of Medicine, Philadelphia, Pennsylvania

KATE MORSE, APRN, ACNP-BC
Assistant Clinical Professor of Nursing, Acute Care Nurse Practitioner Track Coordinator, Drexel University College of Nursing and Health Professions, Philadelphia, Pennsylvania

BOBBIE POSMONTIER, PhD, CNM, PMHNP-BC
Assistant Professor, Dr NP Practitioner Track Coordinator, College of Nursing and Health Professions, Drexel University, Philadelphia, Pennsylvania

MARIAN REIFF, PhD, MSc
Research Associate, Division of Translational Medicine and Human Genetics, Center for the Integration of Genetic Health Care Technologies, Perelman School of Medicine, University of Pennsylvania, Philadelphia, Pennsylvania

JOANNE FARLEY SEREMBUS, EdD, RN, CCRN, CNE
Associate Clinical professor, College of Nursing and Health Professions, Drexel University, Philadelphia, Pennsylvania

MARY ELLEN SMITH GLASGOW, PhD, RN, ACNS-BC
Dean, and Professor Duquesne University School of Nursing, Pittsburgh, Pennsylvania

MAUREEN SROCZYNSKI, DNP, RN
President/CEO, Farley Associates, Norton, Massachusetts; Fellow, Rhode Island Center for Nursing Excellence (RICNE), Kingston, Rhode Island

EILEEN SULLIVAN-MARX, PhD, RN, FAAN
Dean and Erline Perkins McGriff Professor, New York University College of Nursing, New York, New York

ANN MARIE WALSH BRENNAN, PhD, RN
Practice Associate Professor, Division of Biobehavioral and Health Sciences, Coordinator for Curricular Implementation, School of Nursing University of Pennsylvania, Philadelphia, Pennsylvania

DEBORAH L. WEATHERSPOON, PhD(c), CRNA, RN
Assistant Professor, School of Nursing, Middle Tennessee State University, Murfreesboro, Tennessee

TAMI H. WYATT, PhD, RN, CNE
Co-Director, HITS Lab, Associate Professor, Chair, Education Technology & Simulation, College of Nursing, University of Tennessee Knoxville, Knoxville, Tennessee

THERESA M. "TERRY" VALIGA, EdD, RN, ANEF, FAAN
Professor and Director, Institute for Educational Excellence, Duke University School of Nursing, Durham, North Carolina

Contents

Preface: New Developments in Nursing Education: A Focus on Contemporary Content, Pedagogies, Deans, and Trends   xiii

Mary Ellen Smith Glasgow

Nursing Education Trends: Future Implications and Predictions   423

Theresa M. "Terry" Valiga

This article examines current trends in nursing education and proposes numerous transformations needed to ensure that programs are relevant, fully engage learners, reflect evidence-based teaching practices, and are innovative. Such program characteristics are essential if we are to graduate nurses who can practice effectively in today's complex, ambiguous, ever-changing health care environments and who are prepared to practice in and, indeed, shape tomorrow's unknown practice environments.

A Report on a National Study of Doctoral Nursing Faculty   435

H. Michael Dreher, Mary Ellen Smith Glasgow, Frances H. Cornelius, and Anand Bhattacharya

This article reports on a national study of doctoral nursing faculty, including both PhD and Doctor of Nursing Practice (DNP) faculty. Using a national sample of 624 doctoral nursing faculty, we surveyed individuals on a variety of issues, including succession planning, retirement, quality of life as a doctoral faculty member, their views on the new DNP degree, and how they view the future of doctoral nursing education. Study implications for both DNP and PhD faculty are explored and the meaning of the findings of the study for the future are discussed, including new items that will be investigated in a repeat survey in 2012.

The Paradigm Shift   455

Ann Marie Walsh Brennan and Eileen Sullivan-Marx

This article examines current trends in nursing education and proposes undergraduate curriculum changes that are needed to meet the needs and goals of the Institute of Medicine Report: The Future of Nursing, Leading Change, Advancing Health, and The Patient Protection and Affordable Care Act. Curricular changes were developed and implemented during the development of the Affordable Care Act, the Future of Nursing Initiative report, and the Carnegie Report on Undergraduate Nursing Education. The changes will continue to evolve dynamically and are presented here for consideration.

Primary Care Nurse Practitioner Clinical Education: Challenges and Opportunities   463

Maureen Sroczynski and Lynne M. Dunphy

The Institute of Medicine report and the passage of the Patient Protection and Affordable Care Act present significant opportunities for the nursing profession. As the largest group of primary care providers, nurse practitioners are the critical element in the provision of comprehensive primary care, and a critical element to the success of the redesigned health care system. Nurse practitioners can bridge the gap between coverage and access and provide the patient-centered innovative approaches needed. There are, however, significant barriers that need to be addressed. This article presents a framework for creating innovative approaches to the redesign of nurse practitioner clinical education.

Testing Computer-Based Simulation to Enhance Clinical Judgment Skills in Senior Nursing Students   481

Deborah L. Weatherspoon and Tami H. Wyatt

Expert clinical judgment is the culmination of knowledge and experiential learning that includes reflections on immediate problems and past experience. In nursing education, experiential learning is augmented through the use of simulated clinical experiences provided in simulation laboratories. Various simulations have been reported; however, few studies target the effectiveness of experiential learning using a computer-based simulation available to the individual user. An educational intervention based on Kolb's Experiential Learning Theory (ELT) is examined in this pilot study, to determine the feasibility of conducting a future larger-scale research project on the effectiveness of ELT in enhancing development of clinical judgment skills.

Transdisciplinary Simulation: Learning and Practicing Together   493

Kymberlee Montgomery, Sharon Griswold-Theodorson, Kate Morse, Owen Montgomery, and Dana Farabaugh

The Institute of Medicine, partnering with national private foundations, has challenged existing approaches to health care delivery and patient safety by suggesting a sweeping redesign of the entire U.S. health care system. This article explores the historical and philosophic imperative to change health care education to a seamless transdisciplinary model to foster interprofessional communication and collaboration during the formative training years. To improve patient safety and quality of care and reduce medical error, students in health care disciplines will need to be educated together to practice together effectively.

Learning from Business: Incorporating the Toyota Production System into Nursing Curricula   503

Joanne Farley Serembus, Faye Meloy, and Bobbie Posmontier

The faculty at Drexel University decided to investigate a new model to transform nursing education, aiming to produce a new skill set that would serve to improve the transition of nursing graduates from academic settings to practice, to better serve the needs of patients and reduce medical error. Faculty looked to the Toyota Production System (TPS), which has established credibility in industry and health care settings. TPS has demonstrated increased efficiency and effectiveness, reduced cost, and enhanced achievement of stated goals. Drexel University is the first academic institution to incorporate the principles of the TPS into nursing education.

Preparing Nurses to Care for People with Developmental Disabilities: Perspectives on Integrating Developmental Disabilities Concepts and Experiences into Nursing Education   517

Marcia R. Gardner

The argument that nursing curricula have not adequately prepared graduates to provide appropriate care for individuals with intellectual disabilities and developmental disabilities (DDs) has been put forward for a decade or more. This is of concern because the number of individuals with DDs has been increasing at a rapid rate. Undergraduate and graduate nursing curricula should address concepts of care for DDs across the lifespan and develop strategies to provide students with clinically relevant experiences to support development of competencies for care of this population. Exemplar strategies from the literature are described along with recommendations for further work.

Genomic Literacy and Competent Practice: Call for Research on Genetics in Nursing Education   529

Ellen Giarelli and Marian Reiff

This article presents an argument for research on the practical outcomes of genetics education in professional nursing programs. Nurse educators should aggressively conduct educational outcomes research on the translation of genetics core competencies at all levels of clinical practice. There should be a systematic examination of the factors, that influence graduate nurses' applications of concepts to patient care including type of educational preparation in genetics. The best way to improve health is to understand normal genome biology and its relationship to disease biology. Assuring genetics and genomic literacy among all nurses is a crucial task for contemporary nursing education programs.

The Doctor of Nursing Practice Graduate as Faculty Member   547

Sandra Bellini, Paula McCauley, and Regina M. Cusson

This article focuses on the emerging role of the Doctor of Nursing Practice (DNP) graduate as faculty member. Discussion includes historical composition of faculties. Re-evaluation of Boyer's model of scholarship in relation to faculty roles is examined. Discussion includes barriers facing current DNP faculty as well as the potential advantages that DNP graduates may make toward school of nursing faculties. Discussion concludes with considerations for the future of the discipline as demographics and traditional values shift over time.

Promoting a Healthy Workplace for Nursing Faculty and Staff   557

Dorrie K. Fontaine, Elyta H. Koh, and Theresa Carroll

Promoting a healthy workplace in academic nursing settings is vital to recruit new faculty and enhance the work life of all faculty and staff for retention and happiness. When a healthy work environment is fostered, incivility becomes unacceptable, and individuals embrace a culture where all can flourish. This article addresses the imperative of a healthy workplace, with practical suggestions for making the academic setting in schools of nursing one of optimism and confidence where future generations of nurse leaders are developed.

The Experience of a New Deanship for Two Robert Wood Johnson Foundation Executive Nurse Fellows   567

Rosalie O. Mainous and Stephen J. Cavanagh

With the graying of the professoriate, many deans in nursing are moving toward retirement, which provides an opportunity for emerging leaders to move into deanships. New deans move through predictable stages and enjoy a honeymoon, allowing for some mistakes that might not be tolerated later. Early wins are essential in addition to planned changes so as not to overwhelm faculty with change. It is critical to learn the new culture, identify leaders, perform a thorough assessment as the basis for a strategic plan, and be honest and transparent. The ability to mobilize a cohesive, functioning team is critical to success.

Index   575

NURSING CLINICS
OF NORTH AMERICA

FORTHCOMING ISSUES

March 2013
Pulmonary
Cathy Catrambone, PhD, RN, *Guest Editor*

June 2013
Pediatrics
Patricia V. Burkhart, PhD, RN, *Guest Editor*

September 2013
Addictions
Al Rundio, PhD, DNP, RN,
APRN, NEA-BC, DPNAP, *Guest Editor*

December 2013
Genomics
Stephen D. Krau, PhD, RN, CNE,
Guest Editor

RECENT ISSUES

September 2012
Second Generation QSEN
Joanne Disch, PhD, RN, FAAN and
Jane Barnsteiner, PhD, RN, FAAN,
Guest Editors

June 2012
**Future of Advanced Registered Nursing
Practice**
Robin Donohoe Dennison, DNP, APRN,
CCNS, CEN, CNE, *Guest Editor*

March 2012
Tobacco Control
Nancy York, PhD, RN, CNE, *Guest Editor*

NOW AVAILABLE FOR YOUR iPhone and iPad

Preface

New Developments in Nursing Education: A Focus on Contemporary Content, Pedagogies, Deans, and Trends

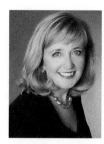

Mary Ellen Smith Glasgow, PhD, RN, ACNS-BC
Guest Editor

We are at an important crossroad in nursing education. The *Institute of Medicine Report on the Future of Nursing: Leading Change, Advancing Health,* released in October 2010, has had time to percolate in our thoughts and is noticeably visible in our professional conversations.[1] With the graying of the professoriate, many deans in nursing are moving toward retirement; it will soon be time for these seasoned deans to pass the baton and share their many years of practical wisdom with their successors so emerging leaders are armed with the knowledge and skills to meet the old and new challenges facing nursing education in the next decade and beyond. What are those challenges? We know that the nursing faculty shortage will be a huge barrier to prepare the numbers of nurses needed for the future. The nursing faculty shortage is an ongoing problem where reasonable solutions with a critical mass impact do not appear on the horizon.

A healthy work environment is one critical solution needed to retain nursing faculty, as well as the encouragement of students to consider the professorial role. If students see faculty stressed, tired, and unhappy, a career in academe will look less and less attractive. Rather students need to observe faculty role models who are engaged, energized, and productive with a reasonable quality of life. To achieve a healthy work environment will require leadership, vigilance, and critical reevaluation of the faculty work life. Difficult questions need to be asked and answered. Is there a place for the Doctor of Nursing Practice graduate in the academy? And if so, is the Doctor of Nursing

Nurs Clin N Am 47 (2012) xiii–xv
http://dx.doi.org/10.1016/j.cnur.2012.07.011   **nursing.theclinics.com**

Practice graduate entitled to all the rights and privileges of the professoriate? What are the salient issues in doctoral nursing education?

It is also a time to reexamine time-honored traditions in nursing education and be open to redesigning clinical education as we face a shortage of clinical sites and faculty. Transdisciplinary or interprofessional models of education are at the core of these new educational models: one that educates nurses, physicians, pharmacists, and other health care professionals together depending on the type of patient needs addressed. But we need to ask, how do we operationalize practicing and learning together in today's siloed academic environment? A solid background in genetics and the scientific basis of health will also be essential for nurses as they counsel patients and truly gain a deep understanding of disease processes and chronic conditions.[2]

This issue of *Nursing Clinics of North America* provides the nurse with an overview of the new developments in nursing education with particular attention to new pedagogies/game-based e-learning, evidence-based care of individuals with developmental/cognitive disabilities as autism rates continue to rise, clinical nursing education redesign, transdisciplinary simulation, a paradigm shift in curriculum from acute care to primary care and public health, doctoral nursing education, and the inclusion of genetics in nursing curricula. New deans will also take the helm at our academic institutions and will need advice as they begin to effect change. Professional work environments will become more important for nursing faculty as the nursing faculty shortage worsens in severity. New curriculum models such as the Toyota Production System will be explored in an effort to teach students about patient safety and heighten their awareness about the need to increase efficiency and effectiveness, reduce cost, and enhance achievement of institutional goals in today's health care environment.

As indicated in the lead article by Valiga, nursing education is challenged with a need for learner-centered environments, diverse student populations, in addition to knowledge exploding at an alarming rate, and a future highly infused with technological advancements, among others.

Although as nurses we may disagree on some of the ideas addressed in this issue, it is important to have an open and honest dialogue about the new developments in nursing education. I welcome readers to reflect on these matters and engage in thoughtful intellectual discourse with their fellow nursing colleagues. The time for change and innovation is now—we need to embrace the tenets of the *Future of Nursing Report* and guide students to lead effectively in today's complex, uncertain, and changing health care environment.

I end this editorial on one cautionary note; we must realize that it may be irrelevant how innovative or competent our future bedside clinicians, advanced practice nurses, or nurse leaders are, if they do not have the ethical framework and moral courage to do the right thing when confronted by the daily ethical dilemmas that are now pervasive in academic and health care organizations. A commitment to ethical practice in nursing education may matter most of all.

Mary Ellen Smith Glasgow, PhD, RN, ACNS-BC
Duquesne University
School of Nursing
600 Forbes Avenue
Fisher Hall, Room 540B
Pittsburgh, PA 15282, USA

E-mail address:
glasgowm@duq.edu

REFERENCES

1. IOM (Institute of Medicine). The future of nursing: Leading change, advancing health. Washington, DC: National Academies Press; 2010.
2. Smith Glasgow ME, Dunphy LM, Mainous RO. Innovative nursing educational curriculum for the 21st century. Transformational models of nursing across different settings. Institute of Medicine Report on the Future of Nursing: Leading Change, Advancing Health. Washington, DC: The National Academies Press; 2010. p. G8–G12.

Nursing Education Trends
Future Implications and Predictions

Theresa M. "Terry" Valiga, EdD, RN, ANEF, FAAN

KEYWORDS

- Nursing education • Educational transformation • Trends in nursing education

KEY POINTS

- This article examines current trends in nursing education and proposes numerous transformations needed to ensure that programs are relevant, fully engage learners, reflect evidence-based teaching practices, and are innovative.
- Such program characteristics are essential to create nurse graduates who practice effectively in today's complex, ambiguous, ever-changing health care environments.

BACKGROUND AND HISTORY OF NURSING EDUCATION

Nursing education does not take place in a vacuum. It takes place in the context of the larger society, the evolution of the profession, and the institutions that offer academic programs. Even the concept of what nursing education is changes over time.

Traditionally, nursing education has been thought of as little more than a course of study, the subject matter taught, the learning experiences that are designed for students, and the collection of courses and clinical hours to be completed. Our early hospital-based education focused more on patient care than on education: schools were seen as revenue streams for hospitals more than institutions of learning, students staffed hospitals to meet patient care needs rather than to learn the practice of nursing, and curricula varied to meet the needs of the parent hospital.

For the past 100 years, nursing education has been the focus of numerous reports,[1–6] and professional associations have issued position statements and/or developed guidelines regarding where nursing education should take place and what its focus should be.[7,8] The accreditation of nursing education programs began in the early 1950s to define standards of quality regarding the curriculum, faculty, and resources. Despite these reports, positions, guidelines, and standards, however, nursing education remained essentially unchanged until what was dubbed the *curriculum revolution* of the late 1980s and early 1990s.

Duke University School of Nursing, 307 Trent Drive, DUMC 3322, Durham, NC 27710, USA
E-mail address: terry.valiga@duke.edu

Nurs Clin N Am 47 (2012) 423–434
http://dx.doi.org/10.1016/j.cnur.2012.07.007
0029-6465/12/$ – see front matter © 2012 Elsevier Inc. All rights reserved.

Through several national conferences and the books,[9–11] articles,[12–15] and conversations[16] they spawned, nurse educators began to think differently about the focus of nursing education, the roles of students and teachers, the ways in which learning experiences were defined, and the ways in which student learning was assessed. Conversations also began regarding the need to base our teaching practices on evidence rather than on tradition.

In more contemporary contexts, nursing education is conceptualized as a means to facilitate student growth; the planned engagement of learners; the dynamic interchange among learners, teachers, and subject matter; and a collaborative experience. There is increasing acknowledgment of the uniqueness of individual learners and teachers as well as the realization that education takes place when the learner's, not the teacher's, objectives are met. In other words, we are moving from closed, teacher-centered approaches to more open, learner-centered approaches to nursing education.

TEACHER-CENTERED AND LEARNER-CENTERED ENVIRONMENTS

Congruent with our nation's historical view of education as a means to discipline the young, provide a moral education, and transmit our culture, educational environments have traditionally been focused on the teacher and what she or he does. Today, however, education is viewed as a means to personal growth, lifelong learning, insight and self-reflection, and deep understanding. **Table 1** summarizes differences between such teacher-centered and learner-centered environments.

In closed teaching systems, teachers view their role as developing only the intellect, preparing students for a job or to pass a licensing or certification examination, and

Table 1
Teacher-centered versus learner-centered education

Teaching Systems	Learning Systems
Powerful Teacher	**Teacher as Facilitator**
• The environment is teacher-centered. • All learning activities are teacher-determined. • The teacher is the authority and the source of knowledge. • Teaching is seen as more important than learning. • Rationality, control, discipline, and an orderly sequence prevail.	• The environment is student-centered. • The focus is on learning rather than teaching or covering the content. • Inquiry, discovery, and creativity are emphasized. • Development of the student as a whole person is emphasized. • Students are helped to learn how to learn and to learn from many sources.
Passive Learner	**Learner as Active Participant**
• The system assumes that only a few students can really learn. • Students are viewed as a collective and not as individuals. • Outside learning is ignored, and only what the teacher presents is important. • All students proceed through the program in the same way and at the same pace. • Students follow directions as outlined by the teacher. • The environment is relatively devoid of feelings.	• Students are seen as colearners with the teacher and with each other. • Students are encouraged to question extensively. • Diversity among students is celebrated. • Approaches to teaching and learning are individualized. • It is assumed that all students can be successful if given the appropriate guidance, challenge, and support. • Feelings are exposed rather than hidden.

passing on our civilization or our nursing culture. There is a specifically designated time for learning, and the teacher structures how that time is used. Students are expected to follow the rules and not ask questions. Failure is seen solely as the fault of the student. Grades and quantitative measures are very important; an emphasis on the right answer predominates. The experience is somewhat mechanistic.

In open learning systems, on the other hand, learning is seen as an enjoyable activity; the focus is broad and flexible; a future-oriented perspective prevails; teachers and students collaborate to determine learning experiences; and there is a recognition that students can learn in many different places and from a wide range of sources, including one another. Affective domain learning and qualitative assessment are seen as important, and an emphasis on the many ways to look at a situation predominates. In open learning systems, students help create the rules and set the pace for the class or course; it is acknowledged that there are many reasons why a student might be unsuccessful; students' life experiences are seen as important; there is a recognition that learning goes on all the time and not just in the classroom or online environment; and learning itself, rather than grades, is the reward.

If there were no other changes in educational approaches, these shifts alone present an enormous challenge to educators. Rather than being in control, teachers in student-centered environments or open learning systems need to step back and see themselves as facilitators (guides on the side rather than sages on the stage) and colearners with students. They need to become comfortable with not covering all the content and with the unpredictability of a class session that is directed, in part, by students' questions, insights, and perspectives. Does this mean the teacher goes to class unprepared or posts a few things for an online course and then walks away, letting the course go where students take it? Of course not, because as teachers, we still have the responsibility to see that students understand the complexities of what it means to engage in the practice of nursing and be a member of the nursing profession. We do not abandon that responsibility. But we also do not need to control or orchestrate every moment of the learning experience.

CONTEMPORARY NURSING EDUCATION

It is clear that education today, in general and in nursing in particular, is moving toward learner-centered environments where teachers are called on to be facilitators of learning. As such changes evolve, it is important to be aware of the context in which they are occurring.

External Reports/Recommendations

As noted, the history of nursing education is rich with reports from external bodies regarding what our programs should be like. Many such reports did not have the impact that the Flexner Report[17] had on medical education, but today's climate seems to be different. Nurse educators are challenged today to respond to any number of recommendations, including the following:

- The Institute of Medicine (IOM) sponsored a health professions education summit in 2002 and recommended at the conclusion of that interprofessional dialogue that "All health professionals should be educated to deliver patient-centered care as members of an interdisciplinary team, emphasizing evidence-based practice, quality improvement approaches, and informatics"[18(p3)]
- After this report, the Quality and Safety Education in Nursing initiative highlighted the importance of adding safety to the 5 concepts promoted by the IOM, and it has become an increasingly significant component of nursing education.

Competencies related to quality and safety have been outlined,[19] and schools of nursing are expected to attend to them seriously as programs are designed and implemented.

- In addition to these quality and safety competencies, nurse educators are being challenged to respond to recommendations from many other groups to prepare students to meet the competencies that those groups deem significant. Such competencies relate to genetics/genomics,[20] evidence-based practice,[21] informatics,[22] and interdisciplinary practice,[23] among others. Indeed, the preparation of nurses for twenty-first-century practice is increasingly demanding and complex, and nurse educators are challenged more and more to focus on the essentials rather than on everything.

- The *Future of Nursing* report recommended that "nurses should achieve higher levels of education and training through an improved education system that promotes seamless academic progression."[24(p4–1)] This education needs to provide learners with "a better understanding of and experience in care management, quality improvement methods, systems-level change management, and the reconceptualized roles of nurses in a reformed health care system."[24(p4–1)] Nursing education has been challenged to be competency based[24(p4–30)] and interdisciplinary in nature,[24(p4–34)] instill in graduates a commitment to lifelong learning, and strive to create an increasingly diverse student body.

- In 2010, the nursing education community was challenged by the Carnegie study (Benner, Sutphen, Leonard, and Day)[25] to transform our practices. As noted by others, these researchers made it clear that nursing needs to "unburden overloaded curricula."[25(p8)] They also concluded that 4 fundamental shifts are needed if we are to prepare graduates for the complex world in which they will practice and that we hope they will shape. Those shifts include an emphasis on "teaching for a sense of salience, situated cognition, and action in clinical situations, ... integrative teaching in [both classroom and clinical] settings, ... an emphasis on clinical reasoning and multiple ways of thinking, ... and ... an emphasis on [identity] formation."[25(p212)] Finally, this report noted that "nursing education needs teachers with a deep nursing knowledge who also know how to teach and conduct research on nursing education."[25(p6)] In other words, these researchers tell us that it is not enough to know one's subject matter or to be a good nurse; teachers of nursing also need to know about how people learn, how to design effective learning environments, how to assess learning through a variety of means, and many other areas. Echoing recommendations issued during the curriculum revolution mentioned earlier, Benner and colleagues[25] make it clear that educators also need to engage in scholarly work to develop the evidence on which our practice as teachers can be based.

- Accrediting bodies in nursing,[26,27] as well as regional accreditors,[28] are challenging educators to focus on assessing the outcomes of educational programs and documenting the difference education makes in the lives of graduates and the societies and professions in which they function. Although licensing and certification examination pass rates remain important in nursing, educators are also asked to document graduates' abilities to think critically, make sound clinical judgments, write and speak in convincing ways, influence system-wide change, and improve patient care.

- Boards of nursing (BON) and professional associations also present regulations and recommendations that are serving to transform nursing education. BON regulations related to outcomes assessment, clinical group size, concept-based curricula, faculty preparation, and other aspects of education influence the design and implementation of programs, as well as faculty development. In North Carolina, for instance, "faculty who teach in programs leading to initial licensure as a nurse shall ... before or within the first three years of employment, have preparation in teaching and learning principles for adult education, including curriculum development, implementation, and evaluation, appropriate to [their] assignment,"[29] (21 NCAC 36 .0318 FACULTY). A rule such as this clearly acknowledges the need for faculty to be prepared as teachers as well as in nursing practice. The *Hallmarks of Excellence* promulgated by the NLN[30] suggest, among other things, that faculty instill a spirit of inquiry and sense of wonderment in students, that students have learning experiences in cultures other than their own, that the curriculum and teaching/learning practices be evidenced based, and that technology be used effectively to support teaching/learning goals.

Diverse Student Populations

As the world becomes increasingly smaller and more students have the opportunity to obtain a college education, student populations are more diverse than ever before. No longer are students homogeneous in terms of their backgrounds, ethnicity, experiences, resources, or family support. Nurse educators are challenged to create learning environments that are effective for students whose primary language may not be English, who have already completed graduate degrees in other fields, who have significant family and work responsibilities, and who have varying degrees of access to technology. Such diversity requires different approaches to teaching, more flexible curricula, and varied ways to assess learning.

Knowledge Explosion

Without question, knowledge explodes at an alarming rate; nurse educators, however, continue to struggle to cover it all in our curricula. Rather than focusing on broad concepts that students are helped to learn deeply and apply in various situations, many nurse educators still present detailed information about caring for patients with various diseases. Rather than focusing on integrative thinking, many nurse educators still present information in isolated silos and assume that students themselves will be able to do the difficult work of integrating those facts into meaningful wholes. Rather than focusing on helping students know where to find information, know how to judge the relevance and usefulness of information, and learn how to learn, many nurse educators continue to present information through lectures and slides, identify specific textbook pages to read, and fail to help students develop self-directed learning skills that will serve them well throughout a lifetime career. Indeed, a trend of the future is to decenter content[31–33] so that our time together with students is used more to focus on learning and integrative thinking.

Technology

A recent warning to the higher education community asserted that universities are committing slow institutional suicide if they do not revolutionize their classroom-based model of instruction. Clearly, open-source learning, badges instead of credit accumulation, mobile applications, online learning, cloud computing, complex gaming, and a myriad of other technological advances are serving to revolutionize higher education; and nursing is not immune. The future is expected to be even more highly infused with technology, which is used to enhance learning, to assess what one has learned, to document achievement of program outcomes, to facilitate dialogue about thorny issues, to access experts in the field, to share resources, to provide patient care, to show data, and so on; and nurse educators are challenged to think about its meaning for the preparation of nurses or nurse specialists. This trend is one that cannot be ignored.

New Program Options

Although hardly new anymore, increasing numbers of Doctor of Nursing Practice (DNP) programs are emerging. These new programs challenge faculty in many ways because they are designed to prepare clinicians who can advance practice by engaging in translational science that leads to evidence-based, system-wide change and health policy formulation. Among other things, new program options, like the DNP and the Clinical Nurse Leader, call on educators to more clearly distinguish the focus of prelicensure, specialty, and doctoral programs in nursing; challenge us to clarify the difference between a DNP capstone project and a doctor of philosophy dissertation; lead us to question who the most appropriate teachers are for such programs; and challenge us to contemplate the most appropriate teaching/learning approaches to help students develop the skills needed for each role and clarify their identity as an advanced clinician, a translational scientist, or a discovery scientist.

Accelerated Programs

From fast-paced baccalaureate programs designed for individuals with degrees in other fields to other program options, such as registered nurse to master of science in nursing, registered nurse or bachelor of science in nursing to DNP, and registered nurse or bachelor of science in nursing to doctor of philosophy, nursing education is accelerating the rate at which qualified nurses are prepared to enter the profession for the first time and seasoned nurses are prepared to move into specialty practice or engage in translational or discovery science. The Oregon Consortium for Nursing Education (OCNE)[34] presents nurse educators with an innovative model to facilitate the movement of learners through associate degree to baccalaureate education in a seamless fashion that eliminates duplication and prepares graduates with the competencies needed to meet the needs of the state's aging and ethnically diverse population. Such collaborative models challenge educators to rethink curriculum models, clinical learning experiences, and our overall educational system.

Simulation

One way to provide a more student-centered learning experience is through the use of simulation, and there is no question that the integration of this method into undergraduate and graduate education is increasing. Using low-fidelity simulators, students are helped to learn foundational skills and implement the nursing role in a safe setting. High-fidelity simulators help students sharpen their clinical reasoning skills, enhance their ability to set priorities, and engage with other members of the health care team to provide patient care. Standardized patients (often identified as a component of or variation on simulation) are also being used in increasing numbers to facilitate learning and to test students' clinical abilities. It is clear that manikin-focused or standardized patient–focused simulations need to be realistic and carefully designed and that the *debriefing that occurs after the simulation is perhaps more critical than the simulation experience itself*. Faculty, therefore, need to develop skills of simulation design, know when to intervene and when to let the scenario unfold without intervention, and lead effective debriefing sessions.

Case Studies

As a way to help students more effectively bridge the gap that often exists between theory or didactic learning and clinical learning,[25] case studies, particularly those that unfold over time and engage students with changing patient situations over time, are increasingly being used in nursing education. This strategy also encourages active student participation in learning and supports the exploration of multiple perspectives on patient situations rather than conveying a one-right-answer approach, which is often the case with lecture and multiple-choice tests. Students might also be involved in creating realistic cases to share with their colleagues.

Dedicated Education Units

Dedicated education units (DEUs), like those developed as part of the OCNE model, offer a new way to conceptualize the roles of learners, teachers, and clinical staff during students' clinical learning experiences. As described by Warner and Moscato,[35] DEUs "turn the tables" and put clinical staff in front-line positions as clinical teachers. Students work directly with clinical staff in caring for their assigned patients, and the role of the teacher is to work primarily with the staff, helping them develop their knowledge and skills related to teaching, assessment of learning needs, providing feedback, and formally evaluating the students' performance. Preliminary outcomes of DEU initiatives are promising and suggest this model has merit for transforming nursing education.

Clinical Immersion Experiences

Another innovative model that shows promise for transforming nursing education is the clinical immersion model currently in use at the University of Delaware.[36] Carrying some vestiges of the diploma school apprenticeship model, as well as current residency program models, the clinical immersion approach to education provides students with extended, concentrated experiences in clinical settings where they have the opportunity to feel as if they are part of the staff, develop collaborative and collegial relationships with nurses and other health care providers, and see patient progress (or lack thereof) over time. More widespread implementation of such a model has the potential to truly transform the way in which nursing education programs are structured and delivered.

Concept-Based Curricula

One final trend in nursing education that is worth noting is that of the concept-based curricula. Work done by the faculty at the University of New Mexico[37] is showing nurse educators ways to move from silo-type education, whereby courses are organized around medical specialties like pediatrics or obstetrics, to a more integrated way of helping students learn nursing. Organized around broad ideas (eg, mobility, pain, tissue perfusion), students are helped to learn core concepts in depth as they explore the meaning and manifestations of those concepts for individuals of various ages and health states who may be cared for in a range of health care settings. Rather than learning about children with casts separately from young adults who are paraplegics, the elderly who have suffered a stroke, or the adult who is frozen and unable to make decisions or take action, students learn about the concept of mobility and explore its many forms; such study challenges students to explore nursing considerations that are common to caring for individuals who are immobilized as well as those that are unique to a particular patient population or health problem. Understanding a concept deeply and from multiple perspectives allows for more integrative thinking and effective transfer of learning than learning isolated facts and circumstances, and it is this deep understanding that is needed to prepare nurses for our uncertain and unpredictable future.

TRANSFORMING NURSING EDUCATION

Despite the changes noted earlier and summarized in **Table 2**, many nursing programs still retain old models. In far too many schools, curricula are rigid, lecture prevails, the primary method to assess student learning is the multiple-choice examination, and teachers design and decide all aspects of the learning experience. If we are to prepare graduates for a lifetime career and a future we cannot even imagine today, we must heed the advice issued in the Carnegie report on nursing: "Redesigning nursing education is an urgent societal agenda."[25(p16)] This advice would benefit all of higher education where "the pace of change is stuck somewhere between sluggish and glacial"[38(p1)] and where our academic culture "strangles innovation and reform."[38(p2)] But what might such transformational change look like?

The following are offered as challenges to the nursing education community if we are to be responsive to anticipated trends and if we are to create such trends:

- Create open, learner-centered environments.
- Embrace change.
- Focus more on helping students form their nursing identity[39] than on covering content.
- Focus clinical learning experiences on in-depth integration and learning (eg, about caring for patients in pain or those with electrolyte imbalance) rather than on total patient care.[39]
- Design curricula that are both structured and open/flexible.
- Do not expect all students to do the same thing at the same time (eg, allow for choice in assignments, place students in varied clinical settings so that broad concepts can emerge).
- Focus on broad didactic concepts rather than specific diseases and treatments.
- Provide for true TEAM, not TURN, teaching, which allows students to think about concepts from various perspectives and see how ideas connect to one another.
- Provide concentrated and immersionlike clinical experiences rather than disjointed experiences or those that are "chopped up" into small bits.
- Focus on student LEARNING and THINKING more so than on TEACHING or COVERING (or getting through) CONTENT.

Table 2	
Summary of changes in nursing education	
From	**To**
• Focus on information	• Focus on processes & outcomes
• Apprenticeship training	• Professional education
• Passive student	• Involved learner
• Medical model (body systems)	• Nursing model (patient needs)
• Skill orientation	• Blending skill & theory
• Basics of care	• Broader scope
• Isolated topics & nursing practice	• Integrated concepts & teamwork
• Doing	• Thinking
• Dependence	• Independence & interdependence
• Highly structured, rigid curricula	• Flexible but sound curricula
• Ethnocentric	• Diversity & cultural sensitivity
• Acute care focus	• Community health & health promotion
• Teacher as deliverer of facts & information	• Teacher as enabler
• Education is time & place bound	• Education can happen at any time & anywhere

- Specify entry competencies for each course rather than merely listing prerequisite courses.
- Provide opportunities for students and teachers to learn together.
- Create classrooms and online environments that are open and encourage a lively exchange of ideas.
- Give students a choice of textbooks.
- Keep teacher-prescribed objectives to a minimum and, instead, provide suggested learning goals, which students can choose (and modify) according to their own learning needs.
- Ensure that affective domain learning is integral throughout the program.
- Provide learning experiences that help students see themselves as leaders who can and must influence the future of patient care and the profession.
- Ensure that teachers think out loud and make their cognitive struggles with difficult issues visible to students so students can see how one thinks like a nurse.
- Use measures other than licensing or certification examination pass rates to evaluate the effectiveness of the program.
- Ensure that a spirit of inquiry and a sense of wonderment pervade the learning environment.
- Encourage and, indeed, celebrate differences.
- Embrace risk taking and mistakes.
- Engage students in conversations that address the uncertainty and ambiguity in our world rather than focusing on certainty and right/wrong thinking.
- Challenge students and expect great things from them.
- Base curriculum decisions on evidence rather than on tradition.
- Design learning experiences that help students learn how to integrate concepts/ideas rather than see them as separate or unconnected things.
- Ensure that the curriculum is a gestalt and not merely a collection of courses.
- Flip classrooms and online environments so that the time teachers and students have together is used to engage in dialogue and struggle with the challenges of what it means to be a nurse (or to take on a new nursing role).
- Expect students to be scholars (at some level).
- Provide opportunities for students from different programs (ie, bachelor of science in nursing, master of science in nursing) and different disciplines to learn together.
- Ensure that a culture of excellence exists for faculty and students.

To achieve such transformations, nurse educators need to think outside the box and refuse to accept the status quo or we-are-doing-just-fine thinking. We need to focus on what students have truly learned rather than whether or not they have put in the required seat time. Additionally, educators should consider requiring all students to have extended experiences with individuals from a culture other than their own.

Faculty should be expected to engage in scholarly teaching as well as the scholarship of teaching and learning (SoTL). In doing so, we would continually question the evidence that does (or does NOT) underlie our teaching practices and evaluation methods. For example, consider the following:

Do all courses need to run for the full semester?
Do most courses need to be 3 credits or more?
Must all students go through the curriculum in the same sequence?
Must all students have the same types of clinical experiences?
Must all students use the same textbook?
Why do we require class attendance?
Are multiple-choice tests really best?

As nurse educators, we must challenge ourselves and our colleagues to separate significant issues from irrelevant ones and essential concepts from the need to cover everything. We need to consider implementing true team teaching with nurse colleagues and colleagues from other disciplines, move with great seriousness to develop interprofessional learning experiences, and work diligently to bring classroom/online and clinical teachers together. We would do well to eliminate old-fashioned courses (pediatrics, obstetrics, psychiatry, community, adult health, and so forth) because they are based on medical specialties and not on how we truly approach the art and science of the nursing discipline. Additionally, nurse educators need to continue trends to study, in rigorous and systematic ways, the most effective ways to enhance learning and fully engage students in the educational experience. As we engage in scholarly teaching and SoTL, we will help develop the science of nursing education—the science that will allow us to engage in evidence-based practices.

In essence, nurse educators must be proactive, anticipate the future, and not wait until history tells the story of our times. We must act despite uncertainty, and we must be innovative and scholarly as we shape the future of nursing education. Transformation is not easy but it is desperately needed. The time is now for nurse educators to use our passion, vision, and persuasive power to lead the transformation of nursing education.

REFERENCES

1. Bridgeman M. Collegiate education for nursing. Troy (NY): Russell Sage Foundation; 1953.
2. Brown EL. Nursing for the future. New York: Russell Sage Foundation; 1948.
3. Committee for the Study of Nursing, and Nursing Education. Nursing and nursing education in the United States (The Goldmark Report). New York: Macmillan; 1923.
4. Lambertsen EC. Education for nursing leadership. Philadelphia: Lippincott; 1958.
5. Montag ML. The education of nursing technicians. New York: G.P. Putnam Sons; 1951.
6. Rogers ME. Educational revolution in nursing. New York: Macmillan; 1961.
7. ANA (American Nurses Association). A position paper. New York: Author; 1965.
8. NLNE (National League for Nursing Education). A curriculum guide for schools of nursing. New York: National League for Nursing Education; 1937.
9. Curriculum revolution: mandate for change. New York: National League for Nursing; 1988.
10. Curriculum revolution: reconceptualizing nursing education. New York: National League for Nursing; 1989.
11. Curriculum revolution: redefining the student-teacher relationship. New York: National League for Nursing; 1990.
12. Allen DA. The curriculum revolution: radical re-visioning of nursing education. J Nurs Educ 1990;29(7):312–7.
13. Nelms TP. Has the curriculum revolution revolutionized the definition of curriculum? J Nurs Educ 1991;30(1):5–8.
14. Tanner CA. Reflections on the curriculum revolution. J Nurs Educ 1990;29(7):295–9.
15. Tanner CA. The curriculum revolution revisited [editorial]. J Nurs Educ 2007;46(2):51–2.
16. Ironside PM. On revolutions and revolutionaries: 25 years of reform and innovation in nursing education. New York: National League for Nursing; 2007.

17. Flexner A. Medical education in the United States and Canada. New York: Carnegie Foundation for Higher Education; 1910.
18. IOM (Institute of Medicine). Health professions education: a bridge to quality. Washington, DC: The National Academies Press; 2003.
19. QSEN [Quality and Safety Education in Nursing]. Quality and safety education in nursing. 2012. Available at: http://www.qsen.org/. Accessed June 10, 2012.
20. Consensus Panel. Essentials of genetic and genomic nursing: competencies, curricula guidelines, and outcome indicators. 2nd edition. Silver Spring (MD): American Nurses Association; 2008.
21. Stevens KR. Essential competencies for evidence-based practice in nursing. San Antonio (TX): Academic Center for Evidence-based Practice, UTHSCSA; 2005.
22. TIGER [Technology Informatics Guiding Education Reform] Collaborative. Informatics competencies for every practicing nurse: recommendations from the TIGER Collaborative. Available at: http://www.tigersummit.com/uploads/3.Tiger. Report_Competencies_final.pdf. Accessed June 10, 2012.
23. Interprofessional Education Collaborative Expert Panel. Core competencies for interprofessional collaborative practice: report of an expert panel. Washington, DC: Interprofessional Education Collaborative; 2011.
24. IOM (Institute of Medicine). The future of nursing: leading change, advancing health. Washington, DC: National Academies Press; 2010.
25. Benner P, Sutphen M, Leonard V, et al. Educating nurses: a call for radical transformation. San Francisco (CA): Jossey-Bass/Carnegie Foundation for the Advancement of Teaching; 2010.
26. CCNE (Commission on Collegiate Nursing Education). Standards for accreditation of baccalaureate and graduate degree nursing programs. Washington, DC: Author; 2009. Available at: http://www.aacn.nche.edu/ccne-accreditation/ standards09.pdf. Accessed June 10, 2012.
27. NLNAC (National League for Nursing Accrediting Commission). Standards and criteria. Atlanta (GA): Author; 2008. Available at: http://www.nlnac.org/manuals/ sc2008.htm. Accessed June 10, 2012.
28. CHEA (Council for Higher Education Accreditation). Directories: regional accrediting organizations 2011-2012. 2012. Available at: http://www.chea.org/ Directories/regional.asp. Accessed June 10, 2012.
29. NCBON (North Carolina Board of Nursing). Education rules. 2011. Available at: http://www.ncbon.com/content.aspx?id=398&linkidentifier=id&itemid=398. Accessed June 10, 2012.
30. NLN (National League for Nursing). Hallmarks of excellence in nursing education. New York: Author; 2004. Available at: http://www.nln.org/recognitionprograms/ hallmarks_indicators.htm. Accessed June 10, 2012.
31. Dalley K, Candela L, Benzel-Lindley J. Learning to let go: the challenge of decrowding the curriculum. Nurse Educ Today 2008;28:62–9.
32. Diekelmann N, Smythe E. Covering content and the additive curriculum: how can I use my time with students to best help them learn what they need to know? J Nurs Educ 2004;43:341–4.
33. Ironside PM. Covering content and teaching thinking: deconstructing the additive curriculum. J Nurs Educ 2004;43:5–12.
34. OCNE (Oregon Consortium for Nursing Education). Oregon Consortium for Nursing Education. Available at: http://www.ocne.org/. Accessed June 10, 2012.
35. Warner JR, Moscato SR. Innovative approach to clinical education: dedicated education units. In: Ard N, Valiga TM, editors. Clinical nursing education: current reflections. New York: National League for Nursing; 2009. p. 59–70.

36. Diefenbeck CA, Plowfield LA, Herrman JW. Clinical immersion: a residency model for nursing education. Nurs Educ Perspect 2006;27(2):72–9.

37. Giddens JB, Brown P, Wright M, et al. A new curriculum for a new era of nursing education. Nurs Educ Perspect 2008;29(4):200–4.

38. Kirschner A. Innovation in higher education? Hah! Chron High Educ 2012. Available at: http://chronicle.com/article/Innovations-in-Higher/131424/. Accessed April 8, 2012.

39. Benner P. Educating nurses: a call for radical transformation – how far have we come? [guest editorial]. J Nurs Educ 2012;51(4):183–4.

A Report on a National Study of Doctoral Nursing Faculty

H. Michael Dreher, PhD, RN[a],*,
Mary Ellen Smith Glasgow, PhD, RN, ACNS-BC[b],
Frances H. Cornelius, PhD, RN-BC, CNE[a], Anand Bhattacharya, MHS[c]

KEYWORDS

- DNP faculty • PhD faculty • Doctoral nursing faculty • Survey
- Nursing faculty salaries

KEY POINTS

- This article reports on a national study of doctoral nursing faculty, including both PhD and Doctor of Nursing Practice (DNP) faculty.
- 624 doctoral nursing faculty were surveyed on succession planning, retirement, quality of life as a doctoral faculty member, their views on the new DNP degree, and how they view the future of doctoral nursing education.
- Study implications for both DNP and PhD faculty are explored.

INTRODUCTION

According to the Robert Wood Johnson Foundation in 2007,[1] half of the current nursing faculty are likely to retire by 2016. This cycle of nursing faculty retirements will be characterized by a surge in senior nursing faculty who will retire that will exceed the number of new faculty replacements.[2] Many of these senior faculty members are doctoral faculty as well as funded researchers. These critical positions will need to be filled when senior faculty retire. But as Potempa and colleagues indicated,[3] there is a lack of adequate role modeling, particularly in undergraduate nursing education, to foster pursuing careers as nursing professors; thus, the pipeline to the nursing professoriate is in crisis. As current senior faculty contemplate concluding their formal careers, we need to focus on providing the next generation of doctoral faculty (PhD

Disclosures: None of the authors has a relationship with a commercial company that has a direct financial interest in the subject matter or materials discussed in the article.
a Department of Armed Nursing Roles, College of Nursing & Health Professions, Drexel University, 1505 Race Street, Bellet Building 12th Floor, MS 501, Philadelphia, PA 19102, USA;
b Duquesne University School of Nursing, 600 Forbes Avenue, Fisher Hall, Room 540B, Pittsburgh, PA 15282, USA; c 2900 Copper Beach Lane, Secane, PA 19018, USA
* Corresponding author.
E-mail address: hd26@drexel.edu

and Doctor of Nursing Practice [DNP]) with the requisite knowledge and skills that will be needed to survive and thrive in academia. We contend that the burning questions facing the doctoral nursing education professoriate are as follows:

- Are current academic administrators actively engaged in succession planning?
- Are doctoral nursing faculty satisfied with their current role?
- Are doctoral nursing faculty concerned about whether DNP program enrollment will surpass and negatively affect PhD program enrollment?
- Are doctoral nursing faculty concerned about the effect of the DNP on nursing knowledge development?
- If the DNP graduate is not educated specifically for an academic role, are doctoral nursing faculty concerned about who will teach nursing students in the future?

BACKGROUND

This survey was the first national study of doctoral nursing faculty, and it included both PhD and DNP faculty and some faculty who taught in both programs. The impetus for this study was the surge in the number of new DNP programs in the discipline and widespread concern over how a new doctoral degree could be widely established in the midst of a publicly protracted nursing faculty shortage. Drexel University's Division of Continuing Nursing Education sponsored the first national conference on the DNP degree in Annapolis, Maryland in 2007 and again in 2009 in Hilton Head Island, South Carolina. These 2 conferences included papers from a diverse set of doctoral nursing faculty, who expressed concerns over:

1. Who will teach DNP students if the DNP degree does not prepare graduates for their role as expert educators in graduate nursing programs (largely in advanced practice nursing programs)?
2. With the demand for advanced practice nurse educators to maintain clinical competency to retain national certification, will future graduate Advanced Practice Registered Nurse (APRN) faculty (for both Master of Science in Nursing [MSN] and DNP programs) be marginalized and largely excluded from tenure track positions with their inability to also engage in seeking and securing funded research?
3. With a national and global recession and intense competition for resources, will the need for additional start-up resources for DNP programs cause PhD programs to lose resources?
4. With such tumultuous changes in doctoral nursing education, what is the current state of the quality of life of doctoral nursing faculty?

Although it is not the purpose of this article to explore these topics in depth, these current and persistent questions framed the need to conduct this national survey to determine how these issues are currently affecting doctoral nursing faculty.

The American Association of Colleges of Nursing (AACN) has been firm since 2004[4] and with the 2006 publication of *The Essentials of Doctoral Education for Advanced Nursing Practice*[5] that the educator role is not an advanced nursing practice role. However, Wittmann-Price and colleagues[6] wrote "...to what extent did members of the AACN (composed of research qualified college and nursing school Deans) fully vet the implications for including the executive role as 'advanced practice' but excluding the educator role as 'advanced practice' (p. 166)?

The question whether doctoral faculty who will teach in DNP and MSN programs are at a disadvantage in the tenure system is a real one. Although Nicholes and Dyer[7] reported that some institutions may tenure DNP faculty (likely institutions that are not research intensive), Irvin-Lazorko[8] wrote "Would acceptance of DNP's as tenured faculty illegitimise a nursing department and foster its marginalisation or strengthen the process by augmenting the professionalism that nursing has struggled to achieve" (p. 75)? Meleis[9] in a recent 2011 point/counterpoint in the *Journal for Nurse Practitioners* again confirmed what probably remains the most predominant view in nursing: that DNPs should not hold tenure track positions. Whether this view remains the future practice in nursing academia is another question.

The third question is whether the surge in DNP programs is a threat to PhD program resources. However, what is unquestionable is that in 2011, with fewer resources in higher education because of the global recession, the number of DNP (N = 184) programs outnumbered PhD programs (N = 125); DNP enrollments (N = 9094) outnumbered PhD enrollments (N = 4907); and the number of annual DNP graduations (N = 1595) exceeded PhD graduations (N = 601).[10,11] Although stagnant PhD graduations and declining full-time postdoctoral research fellowship enrollments in the past decade seem to have slowed, there is ongoing concern whether the senior faculty replacements for research-focused doctoral programs can be replaced with the current pipeline of prospective faculty?[12] With the DNP currently being operationalized as a mostly nonresearch doctorate, this trend has enormous implications for our disciplinary knowledge development.

The central question that this survey sought to answer is: with all the immense changes going on in graduate nursing education, particularly doctoral education, what is the current quality of life for the average nursing faculty member who has a doctoral appointment or who supervises doctoral students even if they are not currently teaching in a DNP or PhD program? As mentioned earlier, no survey has yet focused on doctoral nursing faculty experiences. However, there have been other formal attempts to gather this kind of data among nursing faculty at large. For instance, a 2004 survey of nursing faculty in Minnesota (N = 298; 54% response rate) reported that only 44% had confidence in the general direction of nursing.[13]

The National League for Nursing (NLN) produces the *NLN's Annual Survey of Schools of Nursing*, and in their most recently published report, (April 2011), which was administered from October to December 2010, they raised a couple of issues particularly germane to doctoral nursing education.[14] One of the central findings of this report is that the nursing faculty shortage continues (resulting in 23% of qualified BSN and 32% of qualified associate degree (ADN) students. Second, 56% of BSN programs, 50% of doctoral programs and 40% of BSN programs cited lack of faculty as a main obstacle to expanding capacity. Third, among all types of nursing programs (practice nurse [PN], ADN, Diploma, BSN, RN-to-BSN, MSN, and Doctorate), admission to doctoral programs were the second least selective (16%), with only RN-to-BSN programs (6%) being less selective (or competitive) for admission. Whether these data are similar to schools that are accredited by the Commission on Collegiate Nursing Education (CCNE) is another question. From the Executive Summary, only 25% of full-time faculty in National League for Nursing Accrediting Commission–accredited schools have a doctorate; 44% of faculty teaching in doctoral programs are tenured; 33% are not on a tenure track; and 23% are untenured, but on a tenure track. These findings are explored further and compared with the findings from the National Study of Doctoral Nursing Faculty, which is discussed later. The AACN produces an annual enrollment and graduation report (the PhD/DNP data discussed earlier were extracted from this report), but our review of these most recent reports has found that there are only limited data related to the doctoral faculty role.

METHODOLOGY
Study Design

This prospective cross-sectional study used a descriptive survey with closed and open-ended questions, with the intent of understanding the views of nursing faculty nationally about issues specific to doctoral nursing education, doctoral nursing faculty demographics, as well as on succession planning in nursing academia.

Sampling

A comprehensive list of all US universities offering doctoral nursing programs (DNP and PhD) was obtained from the AACN Web site. An e-mail invitation was sent to the department chairs of all identified programs requesting that they and their doctoral faculty participate in a Web-based survey in 2009 (a follow-up 3-year survey is planned for 2012). Participation was voluntary and open to doctoral faculty from academic institutions offering a DNP, a PhD, or both degrees in the nursing discipline. In order to be classified as doctoral nursing faculty, the individual respondent had to have met one of the following criteria: (1) has taught in a PhD or DNP program in the last 2 years; (2) has been actively engaged in doctoral student supervision (normally PhD dissertation supervision or DNP project/practice dissertation supervision); or (3) has been formally designated as a member of the doctoral faculty in a new doctoral program (typically a new DNP program that was set to launch). Responses were anonymous and personal identification information was not requested. Clustering or stratification was not used in the sampling frame. An electronic cover letter that included an explanation of the study, IRB approval, and information on providing informed consent accompanied the e-mail sent to participants. By clicking on the link to the survey available at the end of the letter, prospective participants were able to provide consent and begin.

Survey Questionnaire

We developed a 32-item Web survey, *A National Survey of Doctoral Nursing Faculty and Succession Planning,* to determine the state of nursing doctoral education from a faculty perspective. This was the first national comprehensive survey of nursing faculty who have taught in both PhD and DNP programs to focus on the state of current doctoral nursing faculty and the future with respect to succession planning. Questions focused on faculty's tenure status, rank, years in academia, teaching role, type of university where employed, presence of an administrative appointment, funding history, retirement plans, current salary, views on doctoral education, job satisfaction, history of succession planning, and demographic data (**Table 1**). In addition, doctoral nursing faculty were encouraged to provide qualitative comments on their views of doctoral nursing education if desired. There were many questions that we did not ask, and the team had to make arbitrary decisions about which questions were most important to limit survey burden. Using several rounds of critique, doctoral faculty who were not involved with this study provided face and content validity of the survey.

Data Analyses

Frequencies and percentages were reported for the closed-ended questions. For questions that required participants to rank order multiple items, the final ranking was derived by using a weighted score to rank each item response. Separate Pearson X^2 analyses were performed to ascertain whether there were differences among faculty who were teaching in a DNP program only, a PhD program only, or in both programs, concerning their level of support for PhD and DNP as well as their perception on how the DNP programs might affect PhD programs in the future. The Fisher exact test was used instead of the X^2 if the frequency of responses for a particular category was low and the assumption of expected count greater than 5 in each cell was violated. Level of significance for all tests were set at $\alpha = 0.05$. All data were entered and analyzed using SPSS for Windows, Version 19.0, (SPSS, Chicago, IL, http://www.spss.com/). Two researchers separately coded the open-ended questions for content analysis to identify emergent themes. Two researchers addressed the trustworthiness, credibility, dependability, confirmability, and transferability of the data.

RESULTS

Of the 631 responses, 7 participants did not meet the eligibility criteria or had more than 10% of their responses missing. These participants were excluded from the final analysis for a total sample size of 624. The maximum margin of error associated with the estimation of proportions from the survey responses was 4%.

Professional Profile of the Doctoral Faculty Participants

Because there is no clear definition of who is a doctoral nursing faculty member, we were faced with having to operationalize the question "Who belongs in this category?" **Table 1** represents the professional profile of the survey participants. The final sample included more PhD program teaching faculty (52%) than DNP program teaching faculty (20%). The remaining sample included faculty teaching in both programs (17%), faculty who had not taught in either program during the last 2 years but who were supervising doctoral students (6%), and faculty who were currently expecting to teach in a new DNP program faculty (5%). Most of the respondents were employed at state-funded or public-supported universities (n = 440, 70%) and at research intensive institutions that require faculty to have external funding to receive tenure (n = 303, 49%). They were mostly full time (n = 618, 93%) and tenured (n = 363, 59%) or on tenure track (n = 138, 52%) if not tenured, earning less than $85,000 (n = 203, 33%) or between $85,000 and $105,000 (n = 210, 34%). Some were currently chairs or directors of both DNP and PhD nursing programs (n = 8, 2%), or just a PhD program (n = 62, 10%) or DNP program (n = 70, 11%). Almost a third of the participants held academic administrator responsibilities other than a chair or director (n = 176, 30%). Three of 4 respondents were full professors (n = 240, 40%) or associate professors (n = 210, 34%). Just less than half (n = 275, 45%) had been teaching for more than 20 years although most had taught in a doctoral program for more than 3 years (n = 395, 65%). Teaching experience was evenly split between exclusively teaching graduate students (n = 253, 41%) and teaching both graduate and undergraduate students (n = 252, 40%). In comparison, few respondents (n = 97, 16%) exclusively taught doctoral students. The number of faculty completing a formal postdoctoral training was relatively small (n = 122, 19%), and just more than one-third (n = 238, 38%) had received a National Institutes of Health (NIH) grant as a principle investigator. Approximately one-quarter of the respondents (n = 168, 26%) indicated that they planned to retire within the next 5 years and half (n = 335, 53%) within the next 10 years.

Doctoral Education in Nursing: the DNP and PhD

Participants were asked about their support for doctoral nursing education, the impact of DNP programs on PhD programs in nursing, and the future of doctoral education in general. In response to the first question "Which statement best supports your current

Table 1
Summary data from study: professional characteristics and faculty responsibilities (N = 624)[a]

Variable	Frequency	Percentage
Taught in a Doctoral Nursing Program		
Taught in PhD nursing within past 2 years	321	52
Taught in DNP nursing within past 2 years	127	20
Taught in both PhD and DNP nursing within past 2 years	104	17
Taught in neither PhD and DNP nursing past 2 years	38	6
Does not apply	34	5
Tenured		
Yes	363	59
Not tenured, but on tenure track		
Yes	138	52
Current Rank is Best Described as		
Full professor	240	40
Associate professor	210	34
Assistant professor	112	18
Clinical full professor	5	1
Clinical associate professor	18	4
Clinical assistant professor	15	3
Full-time working in school/university		
Yes	579	93
Director or chair of a doctoral nursing program		
Yes, PhD program only	62	10
Yes, DNP program only	70	11
Yes, PhD and DNP programs	8	2
No	476	77
Other administrator (not director/chair of doctoral nursing program)		
Yes	176	30
Years Taught Full-Time in Nursing Education (y)		
<3	42	7
3–5	32	5
>5	538	88
Years Taught in Any Doctoral Nursing Program (y)		
<3	216	35
3–5	98	16
>5	297	49
Teaching Role		
Doctoral students exclusively	97	16
Graduate students exclusively	253	41
Both graduate and undergraduate students exclusively	252	40
Undergraduate students exclusively (but supervise PhD/DNP)	7	1
Do not teach	12	2
School/University Can Best Be Described As		
Public/state-supported	440	70

(continued on next page)

Variable	Frequency	Percentage
Table 1 *(continued)*		
Private nonreligiously affiliated	110	18
Private religiously affiliated	72	12
Completed a formal postdoctorate		
Yes	122	19
At least 1 NIH research grant as a principal investigator		
Yes	238	38
Plan to Retire (y)		
<3	59	9
3–5	109	17
>5	456	74
Current Salary ($)		
<85,000	203	33
85,000–115,000	210	34
115,000–200,000	128	20
>200,000	12	2
Prefer not to answer	65	11

[a] Frequency and percentage are reported for available data for each variable. Some faculty did not answer every question and no responses were left off.

view of doctoral nursing education?", among all participants in the study, less than half the respondents supported both the PhD and the DNP "enthusiastically" (n = 265, 43%), whereas almost a quarter supported the PhD and the DNP "moderately" (n = 139, 22%). Others supported the PhD but not the DNP (n = 102, 16.5%) or supported the DNP "reluctantly" (n = 84, 13.5%). Few respondents believed that none of these choices reflected their view (n = 30, 5%). With regards to the question "Which response best reflects your view if the DNP will negatively impact current PhD resources?", close to half the participants (n = 288, 46%) responded that they were "unclear" whether the DNP would negatively affect current PhD resources. The next most frequent response was that the DNP "will" negatively affect current PhD resources (n = 181, 29%) followed by the DNP "will not" negatively affect current PhD resources (n = 140, 22%). The responses to the question "What best reflects your point of view about the future of doctoral nursing education?" were mostly "optimistic" (n = 435, 70%), followed by "unsure" (n = 104, 17%). Few respondents expressed a "mostly pessimistic" view (n = 47, 7%) or did not think any of the choices described their view (n = 36, 6%).

Nursing Faculty in Doctoral Education

This section of the survey consisted of multiple choice questions intended to show the participants' perception related to supply of adequately qualified nursing faculty and nurse scientists for the future. To the first question "Do you think there is going to be an adequate supply of nursing faculty qualified to teach in PhD programs in the next 5 years?", the most common response was a "No" (n = 367, 59%), followed by "Unsure" (n = 148, 24%), and a "Yes" (n = 107, 17%). To the next question "Do you think there is going to be an adequate supply of nursing faculty qualified to teach in DNP programs in the next 5 years?", half the respondents selected "No" (n = 304,

50%), whereas the rest split closely between "Unsure" (n = 162, 26%) and "Yes" (n = 148, 24%). The third question "Do you think there is going to be an adequate supply of nurse scientists to replace the retiring nurse scientists in the next 5 years?" had a similar response pattern to the second one, with most respondents selecting "No" (n = 406, 65%), followed by "Unsure" (n = 136, 22%) and "Yes" (n = 78, 13%).

Professional Growth and Work Satisfaction

This section of the survey aimed to understand the academic and administrative aspirations of the faculty teaching in doctoral programs. The first question we asked related to work satisfaction was "How satisfied are you with your current faculty position?" Most responded as "Very satisfied" (n = 331, 54%) or "Moderately satisfied" (n = 195, 32%). Some respondents were "Just satisfied" (n = 48, 8%), "Moderately unsatisfied" (n = 27, 4%) or "Highly unsatisfied" (n = 15, 2%). This question was followed by "Rank 1–5 the following items in order of priority (#1 is the most important to you) if you could request them to improve your faculty work life." The weighted scores showed that "higher salary" was the topmost priority, followed by "internal resources for scholarships," "reduced teaching load," "improved climate for intellectual discourse," and "higher quality students" (**Fig. 1**). The number of respondents who chose to rank each item as "most important" mimicked the overall ranking except in the case of "reduced teaching load" and "more internal resources," wherein "more internal resources" received a higher overall rank although only 84 respondents ranked it as "most important" compared with 115 for "reduced teaching load." Next, to understand their view on administrative leadership in doctoral education, they were asked "How confident are you in the leadership of the administrator of the doctoral program you teach in?" Most respondents chose "mostly confident" (n = 392, 63%). One of 10 responses expressed "lack of confidence" in their doctoral program administrator (n = 59, 10%). We were also curious to learn about aspirations of the faculty for administrative positions. To the question of whether they agreed with the statement "I am not an academic nursing administrator but I have aspirations to become a director/chair of a doctoral nursing program," the most frequent response was "No" (n = 275, 49%), followed by "Does not apply, I am already in that position" (n = 173, 31%). One-fifth of the respondents were either "Unsure" (n = 63, 11%) or said "Yes" (n = 52, 9%) to aspiring to be a director/chair of a doctoral nursing program. Almost 10% (n = 52) of the sample chose not to respond to this question.

Weighted % Responses

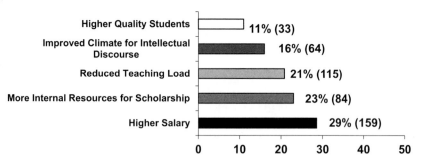

Fig. 1. Weighted response in percentage in order of priority (higher percentage = more important) to improve faculty work life. Number in parentheses indicates number of respondents who ranked the particular item first as most important (n = 604).

Succession Planning and Future Vision

The final section of the survey was intended to address issues surrounding succession planning in doctoral education and their views related to the ability of graduates from DNP programs to lead scholarship and research in nursing through high-quality work. To the question addressing succession planning, more than half of the responses indicated that discussion surrounding succession planning was either "Visible" (n = 231, 37%) or "Very visible" (n = 123, 20%) at their work. Less than a tenth of the respondents indicated there was no discussion about succession planning at all at their work place (n = 57, 9%). When asked to predict "How future doctoral nursing faculty in your institution will view the quality of their work life?" more than half of current faculty believed they would be "Moderately satisfied" (n = 316, 52%), followed by "Highly satisfied" (n = 101, 17%). A mere 4% (n = 25) believed that their work would be "Very unsatisfactory." The final question in this section asked their current view on "How possible is it going to be for future doctoral nursing faculty, particularly those teaching in DNP programs to be tenure track, pursue substantive scholarship and maintain clinical hours for certification?" Most respondents selected "More challenging than it is today" (n = 274, 44%) or "Nearly impossible" (n = 154, 25%). Only 4% (n = 22) believed that the challenges would diminish in the future.

Salary Analyses

Salary data were further analyzed to provide a better picture of compensation in nursing academia based on roles. Salaries of respondents who reported themselves as doctoral faculty only (no administrative role) are presented in **Fig. 2**. Comparison of salaries for department chairs and other administrators is also presented in **Table 2**. Slightly less than half of doctoral faculty (n = 145, 45%) reported an annual salary of less than $85,000. In comparison, as seen in **Table 2**, salaries for department chairs and other administrators were mostly between $85,000 and $105,000 or more than $105,000.

Comparisons Between PhD and DNP Faculty

An important aspect of this study was the emphasis on nursing faculty's support of and perceptions surrounding doctoral education, and the still relatively new DNP degree. Results from the comparison of PhD and DNP faculty and those who teach in both programs about their support for the DNP as well as perception of the impact of DNP on PhD programs are presented in **Figs. 3** and **4**. X^2 analyses revealed that in

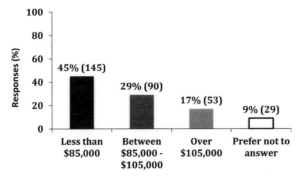

Fig. 2. Salary distributions of respondents who are doctoral teaching faculty only (nonadministrators) (n = 317).

Table 2
Salary comparison among PhD chairs, DNP chairs, chairs of both programs, and other administrators (excludes teaching-only faculty) (n = 314)

Variable (Annual Salary) ($)	Chairs of PhD Programs (n = 62) Frequency (%)	Chairs of DNP Programs (n = 69)[a] Frequency (%)	Chairs of Both Programs (n = 8) Frequency (%)	Other Academic Nursing Administrator (n = 173)[b] Frequency (%)
<85,000	16 (26)	17 (25)	0 (0)	21 (13)
85,000–105,000	13 (21)	22 (32)	2 (25)	33 (19)
>105,000	26 (42)	23 (32)	6 (75)	95 (54)
Prefer not to answer	7 (11)	7 (11)	0 (0)	24 (14)

[a] Salary data was missing for 1 DNP chair.
[b] Salary data was missing for 3 respondents from the Other Academic Nursing Administrators.

both instances the distribution of responses from faculty who taught exclusively in PhD programs differed significantly from those who taught in DNP programs (P<.001). As evident from **Fig. 3**, faculty who taught exclusively in PhD programs were even in their support for PhD and DNP, with more than a quarter exclusively supporting the PhD programs (n = 83, 26%) and almost another quarter enthusiastically supporting both PhD and DNP programs (n = 71, 22%). In comparison, most faculty who taught exclusively in DNP programs provided enthusiastic support for both PhD and DNP programs (n = 96, 76%). In response to the question about the future impact of DNP programs on PhD program resources in **Fig. 4**, almost 2 of 5 faculty members who taught exclusively in PhD programs (n = 123, 38%) perceived that the DNP programs would contribute negatively to PhD program resources. Almost another half of PhD faculty (n = 150, 48%) were unclear whether DNP programs would affect PhD program resources in the future. In sharp contrast, almost half of faculty who taught exclusively in DNP programs (n = 56, 44%) did not think that DNP programs would affect PhD program resources or were unclear whether there would be any impact at all.

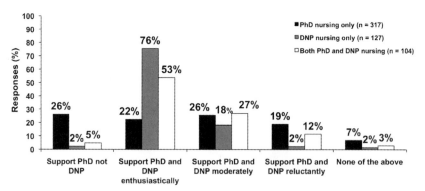

Fig. 3. Comparison of distribution of PhD faculty (n = 317), DNP faculty (n = 127), and those who teach in both programs (n = 104) in their level of support for the PhD and DNP (n = 548).

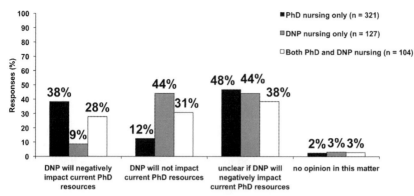

Fig. 4. Comparison of distribution of PhD faculty (n = 321), DNP faculty (n = 127) and those that teach in both programs (n = 104) in their perception of DNP's impact on PhD programs (n = 552).

Qualitative Comments

The following research question guided the focus of this section: "What are doctoral faculty views on the faculty role and the general state of doctoral nursing education?" The focus of the analysis was on both description and interpretation of the phenomena of interest. Five themes were identified for this study: (1) DNP-PhD controversy; (2) déjà vu; (3) research and scholarship; (4) dividing resources and faculty; and (5) respect.

The first shared theme, the DNP-PhD controversy, was based on the many comments that were focused on the tensions between the DNP and PhD degree programs. The following are sample comments:

- I fear the DNP is going to take PhD students.
- The DNP in many schools is turning out to be as rigorous as the PhD and if that is the case, there will be no real difference between them.
- The DNP should maintain its clinical focus.

The second major shared theme of the study was "déjà vu." Most of the participants believed that the nursing discipline had already attempted to have a clinical doctorate and that these new degrees had failed. One comment that showed this view was:

- We already tried the practice doctorate (DNS, DNSc, DSN) only to be discontinued because the programs were similar to PhD programs; however, here we go again.

The third major theme described by participants was "research and scholarship." There was a real concern about who would generate the knowledge for the nursing discipline with the arrival of the DNP. A comment that exemplified this theme was:

- Many of the DNP faculty in our institution are not qualified to generate knowledge and do not value research…. who will be doing the research necessary to move our discipline forward and provide the evidence for evidence-based practice?

The fourth theme, "dividing resources and faculty," described the experience of limited resources in academia and adding a first or second doctoral program. Example comments included:

- If a PhD program is already in place, then adding a DNP program would divide resources.

- I fear the DNP is going to take PhD students, as well as, smaller programs are financially forced to include DNP and PhD students in the same classes.

The final and fifth emerging theme was "respect." Participants described issues with a class system in nursing doctoral education and among faculty. Comments that reflected this theme were:

- The term doctorate applies to DNP, as well as PhD. If clinical practice faculty are equally valued, why are they not awarded tenure?
- Our doctoral council is limited to PhDs. The DNP faculty are disenfranchised and made to feel inferior.
- The issue that is most appalling to me is the opinion of tenure track faculty that a DNP is a second-class doctoral degree.
- Nursing is at an important crossroads. We have an opportunity to generate and translate our own evidence with a cadre of doctorally prepared nurse scientists and a cadre of doctorally prepared practice experts. The question remains how we will operationalize these distinct roles and manage enrollment in both.

These 5 themes have captured the perspectives and thoughts of doctoral nursing faculty related to the state of doctoral nursing education. Doctoral nursing faculty expressed concern about the impact of the DNP degree on PhD enrollment and research for the nursing discipline. There is still a strong sense of uncertainty related to the DNP degree and its impact on doctoral nursing faculty work life and the nursing discipline in general.

DISCUSSION

This picture of the landscape of doctoral nursing faculty indicates that most doctoral nursing faculty in this study were teaching in PhD programs. It is likely that our 2012 survey will include most faculty who are teaching in DNP programs. Overwhelmingly, respondents were teaching at public/state-supported universities. Although most are teaching at research-intensive universities where funding is necessary for tenure (49%), 17.2% were at research-oriented universities where funding is desirable, 16.8% are at research-intensive universities where funding is not required to get tenure, 9% were in academic settings where the focus was more on teaching and basic scholarship for tenure, 6% were at research-oriented institutions where funding is not required, and 2% were in settings where there was no tenure system. With the competition for NIH funding and with resources for federal nursing research funding stagnant, it will be interesting to learn whether the recent requirements for funding for doctoral faculty for tenure will remain the same and, if so, will tenure rates decline? Or, will the tenure and promotion policies of the future be modified?

The tenure rates for this sample were high (59% vs 41%), but of those not tenured (n = 279) fewer were on the tenure track (52% vs 48%). If this trend continues, will doctoral nursing faculty be predominantly untenured and on a nontenure track? If so, this situation would have clear negative implications for individual doctoral faculty and programs in colleges and universities where tenured faculty overwhelmingly comprise the bulk of leadership in the academy; or will the next generation of nursing faculty (possibly DNP-prepared faculty) be sitting around the university/college table? An analysis of our data has indicated that of the 126 doctoral faculty who reported that they were not tenured and not on the tenure track, 39.7% (n = 50) were teaching in DNP programs and 26.2% (n = 33) were teaching in PhD programs; 21% (n = 26) were teaching in both PhD and DNP programs, whereas the remaining 14% (n = 17) reported that it did not apply to them. As mentioned earlier, if DNP faculty members are going to be excluded from the tenure ranks, we conclude that there is going to be another trajectory in the history of the nursing discipline, in which an important segment of the workforce is marginalized.

As for an overall forecast of the future of tenure, much has been written about this recently in the general literature, and we can attest that the hiring of our own institution for recent years has focused more heavily on nontenure track hires, and furthermore, doctoral faculty teaching appointments have increasingly been among nontenure track faculty. At Drexel University's graduate nursing program, the philosophy surrounding the teaching of an individual doctoral course has been more "Who is the best expert and who is best qualified to teach this specific course?" rather than the particular tenure status of the individual.

Salary data from this study have indicated that most respondents had an annual income between $85,000 and $105,000 (34%), closely followed by those earning less than $85,000 (33%). However, this question included individuals who were academic administrators, directors, or department chairs of a DNP, PhD program, or both PhD and DNP programs, and other academic administrators (likely assistant and associate deans and deans). When these individuals were removed, the salary ranges of doctoral nursing faculty in a nonadministrative role (n = 317) were as follows: less than $105,000 (17%), $85,000 to $105,000 (29%), and less than $85,000 (45%) (see **Fig. 2**). Most DNP program directors or department chairs had salary ranges that were clearly split between 32% earning $85,000 to $105,000 and 32% earning more than $105,999, whereas most (42%) of PhD directors or department chairs earned more than $105,000, and 75% of those who chaired both programs earned more than $105,000 (although this was based on only 8 individuals), and 54% of other academic nursing administrators (deans, associate deans, and others) earned more than $105,000 (see **Table 2**).

Most respondents had taught in nursing programs formally for more than 20 years (45%), but less than 3 years in a doctoral program (35%). This situation likely means that faculty taught and then advanced to teach doctoral students later in their careers, not at the beginning. This finding might also reflect the large number of new DNP programs and the possibility that numerous faculty who may have previously taught MSN students now teach DNP students. However, longevity in teaching is clearly related to plans for retirement. Some 53% of current doctoral faculty intended to retire in the next 10 years and another 24% between 10 and 15 years. This finding raises many concerns if the pipeline for not just nursing faculty but also doctoral nursing faculty (often the most senior faculty) is not replenished.

Enthusiasm for the DNP degree (still a relatively new doctorate) was at 43%, but when combined with "moderately" (22%), that percentage increased to 65%. Still, many (30%) do not support the DNP or only support it reluctantly. Of the 231 faculty (37%) who reported that they taught in a DNP program (or taught in both DNP and PhD programs), 7% do not support the DNP degree and another 14% support the DNP only reluctantly (X^2 $P<.001$) (see **Fig. 3**). This finding raises an ethical issue of an individual faculty member who is teaching in a program with which they philosophically disagree or that they do not support. This finding has significant implications, particularly when doctoral workload has to be distributed equally. The merit of assigning faculty to teach courses or supervise DNP projects or practice dissertations (whatever the final work product is called) might be questioned, especially when their motivations to teach and advise these students may lack enthusiasm.

The question of resources indicates that there are differing points of view between DNP and PhD faculty. Among PhD faculty, 38% do believe that DNP programs will affect PhD resources, but among DNP faculty only 9% agree. Perhaps faculty who teach in both programs may be more objective, and of these, 28% agree (X^2 $P<.001$) (see **Fig. 4**). However, there is greater unanimity that it is unclear whether the DNP degree will negatively affect PhD program resources because 48% of PhD faculty, 44% of DNP faculty, and 38% of faculty teaching in both programs agree (X^2 $P<.001$). With a surge in DNP programs, it is difficult to imagine that in institutions where there are both programs, PhD program resources have not been affected, especially with the decline in higher education funds and university and departmental budget cuts. This question does need more investigation and its effect on the discipline, if this supposition is true, needs to be ascertained.

The professional growth and work satisfaction section of the survey indicated that more than half (54%) of doctoral nursing faculty are very satisfied with their current faculty position and, when "moderately satisfied" responses are included (32%), the level of satisfaction increases to 86%, which is extremely high. This number is comparable with the 70% who are mostly optimistic about the future of doctoral nursing education (vs the 25% who are either ambivalent or pessimistic). When a separate analysis was performed between programs, the percentage of those teaching in PhD programs who responded "very satisfied" was 56% and the percentage of those teaching in DNP programs was 52%. For those teaching in both programs, the percentage was 57%. These numbers across programs seem consistent, but overall they do not seem to be exceptionally high. When these same faculty were queried about how future doctoral nursing faculty in their own institutions will view the quality of their work life, the 54% ("very satisfied") decreases to 17%, and the 86% ("very" and "moderately" satisfied) decreases to 69%. This finding indicates that the current doctoral nursing faculty do not think that future doctoral nursing faculty will have the same quality of work life that they currently enjoy.

Fig. 1 indicates that 29% of doctoral faculty rank higher salaries as their chief concern, followed by more internal resources for scholarship (23%) and a reduced teaching workload (21%). Salary issues are well known among nursing faculty, but what constitutes "internal resources for scholarship" is unclear. Although the investigators of this survey considered that this item might include grantsmanship support, editing services, and adequate travel support to professional meetings, for example, it is clear that individual respondents may have believed that this meant something different. For this reason, the 2012 survey will specifically follow up on this question.

Most faculty members (63%) felt very confident in their PhD or DNP department chairs, but no questions were asked about their confidence in the senior leadership (ie, deans) in their college or school of nursing. This item will be included in the 2012 survey. What is perhaps disturbing is that only 20% of doctoral faculty indicated that a discussion of succession planning was taking place in a very visible way in their departments. With the data in this survey indicating that some 26% of doctoral faculty plan to retire within the next 5 years and 53% within the next 10 years, succession planning ought to be a higher priority. Of even greater concern is that only 9% of respondents had any interest in becoming a director or chair of a doctoral program. Furthermore, where are the leadership development programs for the doctoral faculty who could be identified and prepared to assume these roles? Moreover, with the decline in tenure track hires in most nursing schools, will directors and department chairs of the future be nontenure track faculty? This is likely to be a trend among DNP program directors and chairs if they are going to be institutionally classified as nontenure track faculty. Again, if the PhD chair is tenured and the DNP chair is not, what kind of signal does this send to the profession? Overall, we are not surprised that so few respondents wanted to be administrators. Unless there are real tangible benefits to being an academic nursing administrator (and we are aware of many schools of nursing that give these individuals only modest stipends), most doctoral faculty may prefer the flexibility of their full-time teaching roles.

Perhaps our greatest concern arising from the findings in this survey was the percentage of respondents who believed that it would be more challenging than it is currently (44%) or nearly impossible (25%) for future doctoral faculty, particularly those teaching in DNP programs, to have the time to pursue substantive scholarship to achieve success on the tenure track and maintain the requisite number of hours for certification. Combined, this number is 69%, which is a pessimistic view among current PhD and DNP faculty. This finding is of particular concern because, as mentioned earlier, there are now more DNP programs, students, and graduations compared with PhD programs. Will these trends affect nursing academia? Who will comprise most nursing faculty in the future? Is it likely that DNP faculty will constitute the ranks of doctoral nursing faculty teaching in DNP programs? Based on numbers, will the DNP degree become more common than the PhD in academia? Already the AACN indicates that in 2009 to 2010, 24% of DNP graduates were employed in a nursing faculty position.[15] In 2009, Zungolo[16] reported this number was more than 30% and reiterated that these graduates were not being formally prepared for the faculty role because the AACN does not allow DNP educator tracks, nor does it support educator courses that are part of a normal DNP practice or executive role curriculum. The CCNE has also stated they will not accredit such programs. The migration of many DNP graduates into academia, and maybe not solely into DNP graduate education (some are teaching in undergraduate programs too), is a trend that must be studied and addressed. The prospect of a replacement of the PhD with the DNP in academia seems to be a possibility.

The qualitative comments from the survey indicated that there remain barriers between PhD faculty and DNP faculty. Even the quantitative data in this study supported the qualitative findings that the DNP is reluctantly accepted by a significant percentage of current doctoral faculty, and thus the ongoing DNP- PhD controversy has resulted in tension among faculty. The idea of déjà vu (that we have already been down this path) was a common one. With a discipline with several doctorates that have failed the test of time, including the DNSc, DSN, DNS, and ND, there remains concern that this new doctorate, the DNP, may also fail. However, what makes the DNP different from these other degrees is the enormous surge in number of programs. This large number of programs however, does not necessarily equate with impact. Partly for this reason, the recent 2010 Institute of Medicine report on nursing, *The Future of Nursing: Leading Change, Advancing Health*,[17] did not discuss the DNP degree because the panel indicated that there was too little outcome on the degree to make formal comments. Moreover, no major advanced practice nursing organization of practicing APRNs has endorsed the DNP degree as a permanent replacement for the MSN for APRN practice degrees in the future, even although the AACN had called for this transition to take place by 2015 early as January 2004.[18]

From the qualitative comments, there also appeared to be concern over the nature of research and scholarship by DNP graduates. This subject remains an ongoing debate in the discipline. Comments indicated that PhD graduates believe that DNP graduates do not value research and scholarship, whereas some DNPs who are engaged in practice knowledge development or who want to perform clinical research find that their efforts are demeaned or marginalized. Wittmann-Price and colleagues[6] wrote about the kinds of limitations and restrictions that 1 DNP graduate in academia experienced in her new faculty role. Their chief recommendation is that any new faculty member (no matter their degree) needs to fully negotiate their contract and the details of the faculty role, including expectations about teaching, practice, and scholarship, before accepting a faculty position.

The last 2 qualitative responses were related to dividing resources and respect. Again, the fears surrounding resources paralleled the quantitative findings of our survey. A total of 29% of respondents believed that DNP programs would harm PhD resources, and 75% believed that this was true or that they were at least uncertain if this were true. Some even stated that the strain on resources would cause PhD and DNP programs to combine some of their courses. Others believed that the DNP would harm PhD enrollment. Our view is that although PhD graduations are still up slightly,[15] compared with DNP graduations, the PhD is no longer the preferred doctoral degree for nurses seeking a doctorate.

The last theme was "respect." The number of negative comments that DNP faculty had received was troublesome. Many DNP faculty expressed feelings about being marginalized in their faculty role and treated as second-class citizens, particularly by fellow PhD faculty. We are curious whether this trend will continue with our 2012 survey, and we are making efforts to make sure that each of our 5 qualitative themes is explored further.

IMPLICATIONS

The questions posed at the beginning of this article and the results of this study provide insights and direction for further action and inquiry. Priority concerns include: (1) adequate succession planning is absent in many doctoral nursing programs; (2) new approaches to faculty recruitment and retention are required; (3) preparation of the next generation of doctoral nursing faculty is a priority; (4) the role of the DNP in research and scholarship needs clarification; (5) the impact of DNP on the profession must be studied; and (6) trends in tenure may change the academic environment.

Succession Planning

Succession planning is a priority for nursing academia. If we are to be prepared to face the challenges of the future, it is imperative that succession planning be focused and strategic. As indicated, only slightly more than half (57%) indicated that there was any visible succession planning. To sustain and support growth in the future, administrative leadership not only must be transparent in these discussions but also must have in place a structured leadership development program to help faculty grow into future roles. In-house talent development is a cost-effective process for transferring power and authority and should be viewed by administrators as an investment in the future.[19] This concept of succession planning is well established in the business world and should not be foreign to academia. All colleges and universities have strategic plans to guide the institution in a direction aligned with its mission, so why not also put into place processes that will ensure that the right person is in the right position? This subject is relevant not only for faculty in administrative and leadership positions but also for faculty at all levels. In particular, doctorally prepared faculty should serve as leaders and mentors in support of research and scholarship. It is hoped that the 2012 survey will reflect increased attention to this matter.

Faculty Recruitment and Retention

Faculty recruitment and retention is influenced by many factors. The top 3 concerns identified by those surveyed were: (1) higher salary, (2) more internal resources for scholarship, and (3) reduced teaching load. Although higher salary was ranked the highest concern, less than one-third (29%) chose it. Resources for scholarship and reduced teaching load were a close second and third (23% and 21%, respectively), indicating that work-life factors are important. This finding is supported by a recent study of tenured faculty conducted by Berent and Anderko,[20] which determined that to retain faculty, "universities must consider strategies to create a positive work environment that supports the importance and value of the nurse faculty role" (p. 203). This goal includes providing not only a positive and enjoyable educational environment but also providing opportunities for fulfillment, a sense of being valued, and shaping nursing practice. Further research pertaining to all nursing faculty (tenured and nontenured) is indicated to understand job satisfiers and retention factors better and to ensure that qualified faculty are available in the future.[20,21]

The Next Generation of Faculty

We are an aging demographic, with half of the current nursing faculty likely to retire by 2016.[1] Where will the next generation of faculty come from? Will they be adequately prepared to meet the challenges of the faculty role? Trends are indicating that a significant proportion of DNP graduates are assuming faculty positions, yet they are not being formally prepared for the faculty role.[15,16] Given the current and projected faculty shortage,[14] and because more DNPs are being produced, it can be reasonably expected that this trend will continue. This phenomenon must be studied and addressed. If the number of DNPs assuming faculty roles remains stable or continues to grow, as educators, we have an ethical responsibility to prepare our graduates for all future roles that they could be assuming. It is short-sighted not to do so, because this strategy will have far-reaching, long-term ripple effects on nursing education.

Research and Scholarship of the DNP

Research and scholarship are a priority for nursing at all levels of practice. Nursing must seize all available opportunities to generate and translate our own evidence.[2] Survey responses indicating that DNPs are perceived as not qualified to generate knowledge and that they do not value research are troubling. Is this a valid perception of the DNP? Is there a gap in DNP education across the board? More attention to this topic is warranted and may be informed by further study of the impact of the DNP. Dreher[22] has indicated that the DNP graduate must become the leader in producing "practice knowledge" and suggests that the DNP curriculum should reflect skills to enable DNP students to generate practice evidence that will lead to practice knowledge.

Impact of the DNP

An important area for inquiry includes further study of the impact of the DNP on the profession. We must have outcome data. As noted earlier, the enormous surge in the number of programs does not equate to impact. The impact of the DNP on patient outcomes, health care organizations, and nursing education and practice must be studied and documented. This strategy will not only validate the degree both inside and outside the profession but it may also inform the discussion surrounding the DNP degree as a replacement for the MSN for APRN practice in the future. The qualitative responses related to dividing resources and lack of respect reflect the importance of further study of the impact of the DNP. We may find that the contributions of the DNP outweigh the costs associated with dividing resources.

Trends in Tenure

As shown in **Table 1**, the tenure and tenure track rates (including those tenured) for this sample were high (59% and 81%, respectively). However, this finding does not indicate current trends in academia. From 1975 to 2007, the number of faculty who are tenured or on a tenure track decreased from 57% to 31%.[23] This trend is likely to persist because there are cost-saving benefits and increased organizational flexibility, and recent surveys have indicated that most college and university presidents favor faculty contracts over tenure.[24,25] This development will have an impact on the academic environment. It may also have an impact on perception of the legitimacy of the DNP and have a leveling effect within the faculty hierarchy. It is unlikely it will put to rest the DNP-PhD controversy, but it is sure to change the game.

SUMMARY

The findings from this first survey have left us with unanswered questions and have produced additional questions and considerations that warrant further study and that will be incorporated into the 2012 survey. Doctoral nursing education is at a crossroads and is being presented with a unique opportunity to shape the future of the profession. Fortified with a cadre of doctorally prepared nurse researchers/scientists and doctorally prepared practice experts, we have enormous potential to contribute to nursing knowledge and influence nursing education and practice.[2] We have been down this path before. We must take the lessons learned from the past to forge a bold new future for nursing.

REFERENCES

1. Robert Wood Johnson Foundation. Charting nursing's future. 2007. Available at: http://www.rwjf.org/files/publications/other/nursingfuture4.pdf. Accessed June 3, 2012.
2. Smith Glasgow ME, Dreher HM. The future of oncology nursing science: who will generate the knowledge? Oncol Nurs Forum 2010;37(4):393–6.
3. Potempa KM, Redman RW, Anderson CA. Capacity for the advancement of nursing science: issues and challenges. J Prof Nurs 2008;24(6):329–36.
4. American Association of Colleges of Nursing (AACN). AACN position statement on the practice doctorate in nursing October 2004. 2004. Available at: http://www.aacn.nche.edu/DNP/pdf/DNP.pdf. Accessed June 3, 2012.
5. American Association of Colleges of Nursing. Essentials of doctoral education for advanced nursing practice. 2006. Available at: http://www.aacn.nche.edu/DNP/pdf/Essentials.pdf. Accessed June 3, 2012.
6. Wittmann-Price R, Waite R, Woda D. The role of the educator. In: Dreher HM, Smith Glasgow ME, editors. Role development in doctoral advanced nursing practice. New York: Springer; 2011. p. 161–76.
7. Nicholes RH, Dyer J. Is eligibility for tenure possible for the Doctor of Nursing Practice-prepared faculty? J Prof Nurs 2012;28(1):13–7.
8. Irvin-Lazorko PA. I am the doctor: conflicts and tensions of a professional doctorate as a labour market qualification. Work Based Learning e-Journal 2011;2(1):65–82. Available at: http://wblearning-ejournal.com/currentIssue/E3007%20rtb.pdf. Accessed April 14, 2012.
9. Meleis AI. Should DNPs occupy tenure track faculty positions? Rationale against. J Nurse Pract 2011;7(4):280–1.
10. American Association of Colleges of Nursing. (AACN). New AACN data show an enrollment surge in baccalaureate and graduate programs amid calls for more highly educated nurses. 2012. Available at: http://www.aacn.nche.edu/news/articles/2012/enrollment-data. Accessed April 14, 2012.
11. Altundemir ME. The impact of the financial crisis on American public universities. Int J Bus Soc Sci 2012;3(8):190–8.

12. Dreher HM, Rundio A. Education for advanced practice–The "Big Tent" for educating advanced practice nurses: issues surrounding MSN, DNP, and PhD preparation. In: Joel's L, editor. Advanced practice nursing: essentials for role development. 3rd edition. Philadelphia: FA Davis; in press.
13. Disch J, Edwardson S, Adwan J. Nursing faculty satisfaction with individual, institutional, and leadership factors. J Prof Nurs 2004;20(5):323–32.
14. National League for Nursing. NLN's Annual Survey of Schools of Nursing 2009-2010: executive summary. Available at: http://www.nln.org/research/slides/exec_summary_0910.pdf. Accessed June 3, 2012.
15. Fang D, Tracy C, Bednash GD. 2009-2010 enrollments and graduations in baccalaureate and graduate programs in nursing. Washington, DC: American Association of Colleges of Nursing; 2010.
16. Zungolo E. The DNP and the faculty role: issues and challenges. Paper presented at the Second National Conference on the Doctor of Nursing Practice: the dialogue continues.... Hilton Head Island, March 24–27, 2009.
17. Institute of Medicine. The future of nursing: leading change, advancing health, Committee on the Robert Wood Johnson Foundation initiative on the future of nursing, at the Institute Of Medicine. Washington, DC: National Academies Press; 2010.
18. American Association of Colleges of Nursing (AACN). AACN draft position statement on the practice doctorate in nursing January 2004. Washington, DC: AACN; 2004.
19. Clunies JP. Benchmarking succession planning and executive development in higher education: is the academy ready now to employ these corporate paradigms? 2004. Available at: http://www.academicleadership.org/148/benchmarking_succession_planning_executive_development_in_higher_education/. Accessed May 6, 2012.
20. Berent GR, Anderko L. Solving the nurse faculty shortage: exploring retention issues. Nurse Educ 2011;36(5):203–7.
21. Riccio S. Talent management in higher education: developing emerging leaders within the administration at private colleges and universities. 2010: educational administration: theses, dissertations, and student research. Paper 34. Available at: http://digitalcommons.unl.edu/cehsedaddiss/34. Accessed May 6, 2012.
22. Dreher HM. Seeking evidence: practice knowledge development in the Doctor of Nursing Practice degree. Clinical Scholars Review 2011;4(1):51–2.
23. Wilson R. Tenure, RIP: what the vanishing status means for the future of education. Chron High Educ 2010. Available at: http://chronicle.com/article/Tenure-RIP/66114/. Accessed May 6, 2012.
24. Fogg P. Presidents favor scrapping tenure. Chron High Educ 2005;52(11):A31.
25. Stripling J. Most presidents prefer no tenure for majority of faculty. Chron High Educ 2011. Available at: http://chronicle.com/article/Most-Presidents-Favor-No/127526/. Accessed May 6, 2012.

The Paradigm Shift

Ann Marie Walsh Brennan, PhD, RN[a],
Eileen Sullivan-Marx, PhD, RN, FAAN[b],*

KEYWORDS

- Nursing education • Health care reform • Primary care • Health promotion
- Leadership

KEY POINTS

- This article examines current trends in nursing education and proposes undergraduate curriculum changes that are needed to meet the needs and goals of the Institute of Medicine Report: The Future of Nursing, Leading Change, Advancing Health, and The Patient Protection and Affordable Care Act (ACA).
- Curricular changes were developed and implemented during the development of the Affordable Care Act, the Future of Nursing Initiative report, and the Carnegie Report on Undergraduate Nursing Education.

INTRODUCTION

The Patient Protection and Affordable Care Act (ACA) was passed by the US Congress in 2010, and its provision for insurance coverage was upheld as constitutional by the US Supreme Court in 2012.[1,2] However, the US Supreme Court determined that the Medicaid expansion component of the ACA was not constitutional and limited the ability of the Secretary of Health and Human Services to restrict funding to states for Medicaid funding noncompliance with Medicaid.[1,2]

Overall, the main tenets of the Act are to increase the number of Americans who can receive health care insurance and be covered for more health care services, address health care cost through promotion of innovations in health care delivery systems, and prepare a health professional workforce to be able to provide high-quality and valuable health care services with an emphasis on health promotion, disease prevention, and community-based care.[3]

As the nation sees more individuals obtain health insurance coverage either through employers or with public sector funds, including Medicaid and Medicare, the nursing

[a] Division of Biobehavioral and Health Sciences, School of Nursing University of Pennsylvania, 354 Claire M. Fagin Hall 418 Curie Boulevard, Philadelphia, PA 19104-4217, USA; [b] New York University college of Nursing, 726 Broadway, 10th Floor, New York, NY 10003, USA
* Corresponding author.
E-mail address: esm8@nyu.edu

Nurs Clin N Am 47 (2012) 455–462
http://dx.doi.org/10.1016/j.cnur.2012.09.001

profession and supportive partners with the Robert Wood Johnson Foundation and the Institute of Medicine conducted the Future of Nursing: Leading Change, Advancing Health,[4] a thorough study in 2010 and 2011 of nursing, identifying key recommendations for nurses and the nation to address so that nurses are best positioned and prepared to meet the challenges ahead.

These recommended messages include:

1. Nurses should practice to the full extent of their education and training
2. Nurses should achieve higher levels of education and training through an improved education system that promotes seamless academic progression
3. Nurses should be full partners, with physicians and other health professionals, in redesigning health care in the United States
4. Effective workforce planning and policy making require better data collection and improved information[4(pp29−33)]

So what are the challenges for undergraduate nursing education given these reports and recommendations? From the perspective of the Affordable Care Act, more Americans will have access to health care services, increasing the volume of services and the need for more nurses. The US Department of Health Resources and Services Administration estimates there will be a shortage of one million registered nurses by 2025,[5] although some recent trends indicate that newly prepared nurses from younger age groups are entering the workforce in rates that may change this projection.[6] Nonetheless, an expected shortage at any level, combined with increasing numbers of individuals eligible for coverage, will require the engagement of nursing with innovations and community-based services that will be supported by the private and public payers who seek solutions to costly and inefficient care, focusing on high-quality services to achieve such efficiencies. For example, those who have the current highest cost of health care services are those who are covered by both Medicare and Medicaid, that is, they are dually eligible for coverage (commonly referred to as *dual eligibles*). Those who are dually eligible are more likely to live in institutions if older than 65 years.[1,2] Because this is a group with more chronic illness, comorbidities, and functional impairment, costs are high because of frequent hospitalization, emergency department visits, and long-term care needs.[7]

As a result, nurses will be expected to have skills that emphasize community and public health care, health promotion, disease prevention, rehabilitation care, and care coordination so that care between settings is comprehensive, continuous, and seamless. Care will take place in the home, ambulatory clinics, private offices, retail stores, and traditional hospitals, although hospital stays will continue to be short with pressures from insurance providers. Nurses will be increasingly presented with the responsibility for overall patient safety and outcomes that ensure patients in hospitals will be free of newly acquired infections, pressure ulcers, and injuries. Preventing rehospitalizations and readmissions to the emergency departments will create opportunities for nurses to excel in innovations for care provision but also to take a lead in care decisions at many points in the care continuum.

For example, working with teams and technology, nurses now monitor patients' at-home weights and vital signs from a distance and make early intervention recommendations on care—diet, fluid intake, medication review and potential changes, and physical activity—in coordination with other health care professionals and interdisciplinary teams. Taking these types of innovations and programs to scale and standardizing them not only require that insurance covers such programs but also that a nurse workforce is educated in appropriate critical thinking, ethical approaches, and judgment skills.

Given the Future of Nursing Recommendations,[4] what would the effect be for each? What would it look like to have nursing education address each of these issues?

1. Nurses should practice to the full extent of their education and training. Often this practice refers to the advanced practice nurse role, but registered nurses are highly educated and not always enabled to practice to the full extent. For example, registered nurses as part of a hospital team of care could make decisions about a patient's diet moving from clear to full liquids after minor head trauma. In home health care, the primary nurse could work with the physical therapist and recommend changes in a therapy regimen without waiting for a physician order.

2. Nurses should achieve higher levels of education and training through an improved education system that promotes seamless academic progression. Educators and schools of nursing must create opportunities to articulate across programs to reach a goal of 80% BSN by 2020. Online learning opportunities are underway and could be enhanced, bridging community colleges and universities. Colleges offering bachelor's degrees can make the transition from one level to another more seamless in partnership with national and state boards of nursing. Registered nurses are still most likely to be prepared at the associate degree level.[8] Because of the faculty shortage which limits access to upper level BSN education, registered nurses are still most likely to be prepared at the associate degree level. In addition these types of community college based offerings foster educational opportunities in rural and distant areas.

3. Nurses should be full partners, with physicians and other health professionals, in redesigning health care in the United States. One important area to address more consistently and formally in the undergraduate curriculum to achieve this recommendation is a stronger focus on leadership education for nurses to lead programs and initiatives and manage and work within systems of care. Leadership skills related to policy and organizational development aimed at implementing change and initiating innovation are not as imbedded in nursing curricula as they could be, particularly those skills related to interprofessional interactions.

4. Effective workforce planning and policy making require better data collection and improved information. Educators will need to use data for projections of students and faculty. To better address community-based learning and public health as well as judgment driven care, use of data and technology must become available to policymakers, educators, students, and practicing nurses. How to use data needs to be strongly emphasized in curriculum at the undergraduate level. Creativity in curriculum will depend on knowing the data on which to build and innovate.

As we move forward to address the Future of Nursing Initiative within the context of the implementation of the ACA, educational programs for nursing will address partnerships with the health care providers, systems of care, and communities. Preparing nurses to address health and illness will increasingly take place where people live, work, and play, so bringing community into the classroom and simulation laboratory will be expanded in curricula. We present a case study of change in the undergraduate program at the University of Pennsylvania School of Nursing. Curricular changes were developed and implemented during the development of the ACA, the Future of Nursing Initiative report, and the Carnegie Report on Undergraduate Nursing Education. The changes will continue to evolve dynamically and are presented here for consideration.

CASE STUDY

What does the undergraduate need to meet the challenges in the primary care, health promotion, and public health arenas? How should a curriculum be structured to educate students to appreciate the intricacies and complexities of these care situations and be prepared to implement well thought out interventions for individuals and communities?

The process starts with giving students the basic building blocks for primary care. These tools can be provided in several ways—there is no one curriculum to meet these needs, and every school will want to assess its own strengths and mission to identify not only what each is already doing well but where a refocus will highlight primary care in a way that helps students see the possibilities and motivate them to pursue this aspect of care.

At the University of Pennsylvania, we are implementing a new curriculum that introduces students early to basic content, skills, and tools necessary for success in primary care in freshman and sophomore courses and then, beginning in the sophomore year, shows them how these can be applied. Students move on to work applicable to acute care environments in their junior year but return for a full semester of immersion in health care in the community for the first semester of their senior year. In the final semester students apply what they have learned related to care coordination, critical thinking and ethical and clinical judgment and focus on leadership skills in action in a variety of clinical settings including those based in the community.

Much of what we are doing in our new curriculum builds on the recommendations of the Carnegie Report.[9] There is a focus on contextualizing nursing knowledge to reinforce the salience of the content and, we hope, retention of the knowledge and skill. This focus is most important for primary care and health promotion. There is a need to introduce students early to nonacute aspects of nursing, not just acute care. This introduction is especially important because many students coming to nursing have little conception of nursing roles in anything other than acute care settings, and the desire to work in acute care is what often motivates an interest in nursing.

In this new curriculum, students are introduced early to skills that will enhance their ability to participate in primary care activities. They learn communication skills, including both therapeutic and motivational interviewing, and physical assessment. They learn history-taking skills and how to assess health behaviors. They consider community environments with particular focus on what environmental factors will enhance or be detrimental to health. They discuss health care policy and health care equity and access. They begin to discuss culture and ethnic background as necessary considerations in developing effective interventions. We have also integrated Quality and Safety in Nursing Education (QSEN) (http://www.qsen.org/)[10] competencies at an early stage, with content building in complexity as the curriculum progresses, for example, in light of QSEN's promotion of interprofessional collaboration, second-semester freshmen students heard a panel discussion that focused on the teamwork needed to meet the needs of members of our school-run pace program, LIFE—Living Independently for Elders. That panel consisted of a social worker, occupational therapist, and nurse. These students build on this initial understanding in poster presentations of pertinent aspects of different types of nursing, with interprofessional interaction highlighted on each. Although our school has chosen to integrate QSEN competencies, it may be more appropriate for another school to have a freestanding QSEN course. All of these areas of content and activity are among the building blocks students need to be able to move into primary care and, in our curriculum, are covered in freshman and the first half of sophomore year.

Of these skills, 2 stand out as being particularly important to any primary care effort: motivational interviewing and behavioral interventions. Motivational interviewing is a patient-centered skill set that students can use to promote behavioral change. In primary care settings, this skill can be particularly helpful in promoting health by tackling such issues as adherence to medication régimes or other health promotion behaviors, such as smoking cessation or adapting a healthy diet. The technique assists in uncovering and clarifying ambivalence, supporting the possibility of change, and developing the capacity to plan to carry out a change. Behavioral interventions addressing chronic health conditions also need to be addressed. Students need to be aware of population health statistics and understand the need to develop programs aimed at high impact conditions in a particular community, for example, diabetes, heart disease, or cancer.

Specific curriculum on primary care is introduced in the second half of their sophomore year in a course that focuses on health concerns of women. Although the perspective of this course is both national and global (a focus on the World Health Organization's Millennial Development Goals [http://www.un.org/millenniumgoals/][11] contributing to the latter), most of the clinical experiences are in primary care settings in local communities. The course focuses on health needs and risk assessment of adolescent, midlife, and older women. The adolescent component addresses growth and development screening, immunizations, health screening, and health promotion in the areas of nutrition and sleep. Common adolescent reproductive health and medical concerns, such as acne, abdominal pain, and fatigue, are covered as is helping adolescents with chronic illness cope in the community. Sexual health and gender issues, including health screening considerations for the lesbian, gay, bisexual, transgender, and intersex communities, and partner violence are also covered. Behavioral health screening and substance abuse influence on adolescents are addressed.

The midlife component gains some direction from the United Nations' Pillars of Safe Motherhood (http://www.safemotherhood.org/)[12] and covers common health screening and promotion concerns for this age group as well as reproductive content, including sexual transmitted diseases, contraception, abortion, and healthy child birth. Postpartum concerns both globally and locally are addressed. Infant care, feeding and lactation, immunizations, and participatory guidance for parents with newborns are discussed and practiced.

The primary care focus on older women in this sophomore course also includes health screening, health promotion needs, and preventative care based on national recommendations, for example, related to cancer, heart disease, and osteoporosis. National recommendations for care of perimenopausal and menopausal women are discussed as is the use of complementary health care interventions in the context of perimenopause. Stress, exercise, and emotional and physical demands on women, including in the caregiver role, will be covered. Sexuality and intimacy in older women are also considered. Social and psychological issues concerning older women, for example, socioeconomic status vulnerability, decisions related to driving, living longer than men, loss of a loved one, and grief are also addressed.

Nursing students also need an understanding of health care policy and the Affordable Health Care Act and their impact on community health. Students in our new curriculum are required to take a health care policy course during their junior year in addition to a health care ethics course that had been previously required.

Our junior year is one of acute care focus, and students will use the skills they acquired related to health promotion, teaching, and communication among others. The students will return to focused primary and community care experience in a semester-long senior year course. We believe that at this point students should have developed the skill, knowledge, and clinical judgment for a more independent practice that is needed in the community. We also have a goal that by this time students will better appreciate the complex needs of communities and, therefore, the complex skill set required of a nurse working in the community. A community/ public health course needs to explore the relationship between the nurse and the patient as a consumer. In the community, students need to consider that it can also be the patient/community as a consumer of health care. Students need to consider motivations behind community health requests, for example, when a church contacts a student group to come to them to do finger sticks, students need to explore why the church perceives this as a need. Can this initial access begin a series of presentations related to health, nutrition, diabetes, obesity, and breast feeding as one positive intervention toward the reduction of obesity?

This course offers students the opportunity to consider public health and population-based nursing including the historical development and structure of public health and health care systems for groups, families, and individuals living within particular communities and for the community as a population. Public health core functions and the intersections between the sciences of nursing and public health will also be discussed, as will interprofessional and intersystems practice. In addition to public health, the students will also consider community nursing roles and practice including the complexity of this practice: local and global perspectives in relation to public health, community health, and population health. Sites and roles of community health nursing practice and theory and practice of change in communities are discussed. The students have the opportunity to look at the big picture by completing a community readiness assessment and considering the challenges for individuals and families by managing transitions to, and in, the community and exploring home health care.

Content in the course also includes community-based participatory teaching, practice, and research; public and community health approaches to groups at risk; issues of quality and safety in sites of public health, community care; and technology and health in the community. Communication skills are clearly necessary for success in the community, and students will consider communication as a process of understanding meaning; creating partnerships; respect; and developing, recognizing, and will develop, recognize and nurture their voice and ability to act effectively.

Many students in our program are interested in global nursing and participation with nongovernmental organizations. To anchor this interest, the course includes a global health case study in which students consider health initiatives in an established refugee camp setting. International Congress of Nursing disaster nursing competencies will be addressed (http://www.icn.ch/images/stories/documents/publications/position_statements/A11_Nurses_Disaster_Preparedness.pdf).[13] The students are divided in groups and assigned to address basic needs in the camp, for example, primary health/immunization issues, waterborne disease, nutrition, and mental health, particularly posttraumatic stress screening for new arrivals. A mock United Nations Coordination meeting will be held, and representatives from each group will present their group's findings with an overview of their response plan for that particular problem, identifications of what assessments are needed, identification of who from the community needs to be engaged in the planning, and consideration of ways to integrate the other programs to minimize stress to the community.

The course also returns to concepts introduced in the sophomore year and addresses at a greater level of complexity such things as health equity, immigrant health, global health, and public and community health approaches to violence. Finally, the complexity and accountability of nursing practice across spectrum of emergency management is covered, including preparedness, response, recovery, mitigation and all hazard response.

While primary care, health promotion, and public health content may be part of the required curriculum, there are possibilities for the development of additional electives.

These electives are service-based learning courses that focus on community or, as in our school, the development of what we call a *case study course*, a course that is somewhat like an elective but with a clinical component. In such a course, a small group of nursing students could focus on the primary health concerns of a particular community. In our school, although elective courses and service-based learning courses are open to all university students, case studies are restricted to nursing students because of the value placed on that clinical experience and the need to have the requisite skills to be successful in a clinical setting.

The same questions asked of undergraduate education also need to be addressed by postbaccalaureate programs. What are the key competencies needed by nurse practitioners to address primary care, health promotion, and public health needs? The consensus model currently drives advanced practice education. Students need the knowledge and technical skills necessary for sound clinical decision making. A solid articulation of concepts related to health promotion, maintenance, prevention, and restoration is basic. Laboratory and diagnostic testing needs to be covered to support differential diagnosis. Scope of practice also needs to be addressed so that students are comfortable with their judgment skills to support making referrals when a patient presents with ambiguous or complicated medical situations. Experiences need to be tailored to ambulatory, community, and occupational settings. Interprofessional communication, consultation, and collaboration skills need to be fostered. Skills to critique research in support of a primary health practice need to be developed. Students need a firm grounding in evidenced-base practice. Knowing how to identify quality community services and resources to promote health is also important.

Graduate programs need to build on the baccalaureate understanding of ethical issues, political and policy issues, advocacy for patients and policy, cultural competency, functional status, health literacy, and developmental imperatives and how they apply to primary care situations. Teaching skills need to be advanced. Ability to implement quality and safety standards is necessary.

An understanding of the context of providing primary care also needs to be considered. What are the economic, management, and organizational considerations pertinent to primary care? What are systems challenges? What are the legal and licensure limitations on practice? Do these impact reimbursements? What are credentialing imperatives? What case management skills are required? What peer skills are necessary? How does one evaluate peers, for example, related to clinical documentation? What self-evaluation skills are necessary? How does one evaluate a system with the aim of improving patient outcomes? A core competency of nurse practitioners is community engagement. Nurse practitioners should be able to conduct focus groups with patients, and students should be taught the skills to do this. And what is the bigger picture? What knowledge of appropriate models of care is needed, for example, the Dunphy Advanced Practice Nursing Model of Care?

SUMMARY

This is an exciting time for nursing, one of challenge and potential. Changes initiated by the ACA demand creative responses in education and practice. The curriculum case presented aims at student's ability to provide effective primary care and focuses on competence building earlier in the curriculum with more opportunities to engage with patients to build confidence in performance. Content threads build in complexity. The goal is to have students ready to move forward at an earlier stage, to be able to grasp the complexities of primary care work, to gain that experience in a supportive environment, and ultimately to be ready to move into the future of nursing.

REFERENCES

1. Kaiser Family Foundation. The diversity of dual eligible beneficiaries: an examination of services and spending for people eligible for both Medicaid and Medicare. Washington, DC: Author; 2012. Available at: http://www.kff.org/medicaid/upload/7895-02.pdf. Accessed September 3, 2012.
2. Kaiser Family Foundation. A guide to the Supreme Court's decision on the ACA's Medicaid expansion. Washington, DC: Author; 2012. Available at: http://www.kff.org/healthreform/upload/8347.pdf. Accessed September 2, 2012.
3. U.S. Department of Health, Human Services, Centers for Medicare & Medicaid Services. The Affordable Care Act: lowering Medicare costs by improving care. Washington, DC: Author; 2012. Available at: http://www.cms.gov/apps/files/ACA-savings-report-2012.pdf. Accessed September 2, 2012.
4. National Research Council. The future of nursing: leading change, advancing health. Washington, DC: The National Academies Press; 2011.
5. U.S. Department of Health & Human Services, Health Resources and Services Administration. Health professions. 2009. Available at: http://bhpr.hrsa.gov/about/bhprfactsheet.pdf. Accessed September 2, 2012.
6. Auerbach D, Buerhaus P, Staiger D. Surge in those ages 23-26 entering the registered nurse work force means that supply is growing faster than projected. Health Aff 2011;30(12):2286–92.
7. Thorpe KE, Ogden LL, Galactionova K. Chronic conditions account for rise in Medicare spending from 1987 to 2006. Health Aff 2010;29:718–24.
8. U.S. Department of Health, Human Services, Health Resources and Services Administration. The registered nurse population: findings from the 2008 national sample survey of registered nurses, 2010. Washington, DC: Author; 2010.
9. Benner P, Sutphen M, Leonard V, et al. Educating nurses: a call for radical transformation. San Francisco: Jossey-Bass; 2010.
10. Quality and Safety for Nurses. Available at: http://www.qsen.org/.
11. Millennium Development Goals. Available at: http://www.un.org/millenniumgoals/. Accessed August 27, 2012.
12. Pillars of Safe Motherhood. Available at: http://www.safemotherhood.org/.
13. International Congress of Nursing. Available at: http://www.icn.ch/images/stories/documents/publications/position_statements/A11_Nurses_Disaster_Preparedness.pdf.

Primary Care Nurse Practitioner Clinical Education

Challenges and Opportunities

Maureen Sroczynski, DNP, RN[a,b,]*,
Lynne M. Dunphy, APRN, FNP-BC, PhD[c]

KEYWORDS

- Nurse practitioner education • Clinical nursing education
- Competency-based education • Nursing workforce • Clinical partnerships
- Interprofessional education (IPE) • Health care reform

KEY POINTS

- Health care reform makes the preparation of nurse practitioners more essential than ever.
- The Gap Analysis process provides a methodology to frame clinical education redesign.
- Competency/outcome based models can serve as the foundation of clinical education redesign.
- Current health care reform is creating the demand for a more highly educated nursing workforce.
- Inter-professional education models provide the most direct approach to enhance the quality of care in all health care settings.

The recent Institute of Medicine[1] (IOM) report on the future of nursing and the passage of health care reform present many demands and opportunities for all health care professionals.[2] The primary demands are arising from the need to create a health care system that is patient centered and focused on primary care, care coordination, transitional care, prevention, and wellness. Both the IOM and the Patient Protection and Affordable Care Act have identified the need to increase access to primary care providers as necessary to the success of this redesigned health care system. As the largest group of primary care providers, nurse practitioners (APRNs) are the critical

Disclosures: None of the authors has a relationship with a commercial company that has a direct financial interest in the subject matter expressed in the article.
a Farley Associates, 238 East Main Street, #15, Norton, MA 02766, USA; b Rhode Island Center for Nursing Excellence, 2 Heathman Road, #138 White Hall, Kingston, RI 02881, USA; c Rhode Island center for Nursing Excellence, College of Nursing, University of Rhode Island, 2 Heathman Road, #138 White Hall, Kingston, RI 02881, USA
* Corresponding author.
E-mail address: msrocz@aol.com

Nurs Clin N Am 47 (2012) 463–479
http://dx.doi.org/10.1016/j.cnur.2012.08.001
0029-6465/12/$ – see front matter © 2012 Elsevier Inc. All rights reserved.
nursing.theclinics.com

element in the provision of comprehensive primary care, prevention, and quality outcomes. With the potential addition of 32 million more individuals to the ranks of the insured, APRNs can bridge the gap between coverage and access and provide the patient-centered innovative approaches needed to improve health. Nurse practitioners will be the "glue" of the health care system and will continue to assume a lead role in the quality and efficiency of the redesigned system.[3]

Countries that build their health care systems on the cornerstone of primary care have better health outcomes and more equitable access to care.[4] The Patient Protection and Affordable Care Act is providing approximately $30 million to train additional APRNs to provide comprehensive primary care and more than $5 million for states to plan and implement innovative strategies to expand their primary care workforce to meet the increased demand for primary care services.[5] Although this increase in funding does provide incentives for nursing programs to expand their capacity for APRN education, there are significant barriers that need to be addressed to effectively expand APRN programs specifically in primary care. Faculty shortages, the lack of appropriate clinical placements, and the continuing calls for education reform are placing increasing demands on the entire nursing education system.[2] The dynamics of the country's rapidly evolving health care delivery system, especially the financing, are intensifying the competition and access to clinical learning opportunities in both acute care and community sites. These demands are necessitating creative strategies and new approaches to facilitate clinical learning and experiences across nursing education programs.

Opportunity and innovation are born out of crisis.[6] In the changing health care environment, nurse educators on all levels must take advantage of any and all opportunities to redesign nursing education to continue to prepare the highly qualified practitioners that will be needed for the future health care system.

BACKGROUND

Currently, there are approximately 400,000 primary care providers in the United States, representing 287,000 physicians, 83,000 APRNs, and 23,000 physician assistants.[1] The number of residents entering primary care and family practice are decreasing as the number of APRNs and physical assistants are continuing to increase.[7] The number of adult primary care practitioners overall is estimated to grow by only 2% to 7% from 2005 to 2025. Population growth and aging are estimated to increase the workload of adult primary care practitioners by 29% during this same time period. These estimates are projected to lead to a shortage of 35,000 to 40,000 primary care practitioners.[8]

The primary care workforce as whole will need to increase by up to 25% to meet the demands of health care reform.[9] These figures are validated by other studies.

The numbers of those entering primary care is not seen as sufficient to close this gap. For nursing, the number of graduates in the specialties usually designated as primary care (family, adult, gerontology, pediatric, and women's health) totaled 9203 in the 2009–2010 academic year, an increase of only 752 from the previous year.[10–12] From this perspective, the IOM[1] recommends expansion of scope of practice in primary care and the reform of nursing education to more effectively prepare all nurses to practice to the full extent of their knowledge and competence. This will require removing barriers to the scope of practice of all APRNs across the country and the expansion of capacity in APRN education programs. To meet this challenge, nursing programs throughout the country will need to develop innovative approaches to increase capacity and funding for primary care APRN students.

To meet these educational and workforce challenges, the APRN community has come together to address both the misunderstanding and inconsistencies in APRN roles and education. In 2008, a collaborative of the APRN Consensus Work Group and the National Council of State Boards of Nursing APRN Advisory Committee with input from the larger APRN stakeholder community developed the Consensus Model for APRN Licensure, Accreditation, Certification, and Education to address the lack uniformity in educational and state regulations. This document in combination with the Carnegie report on educating nurses[2] and the IOM[1] report on the future of nursing provides the framework for development of the innovative approaches needed to strengthen APRN education and ensure a continuing supply of high-quality primary care APRNs.

APPROACH

The approach to this topic includes (1) a gap analysis framework to guide inquiry, (2) a literature review to identify current trends in primary nursing and medical education models, and (3) identification of competencies and outcomes that are common to the new models.

GAP ANALYSIS

To begin, we used a gap analysis approach. This approach involves a comparative study of the present state and the desired or future state This process begins with the listing of the characteristic factors (standards, regulations, competencies) of the present state (what is) with a cross-listing of factors required to achieve future objectives (what could be) and then highlighting the gaps that exist and need to be filled.[13,14] Both the Massachusetts Nurse of the Future project and the Quality and Safety Education for Nurses project included similar processes. A set of guiding questions is often used to frame the process. The guiding questions for this work included:

- What are the standards for APRN clinical education in primary care?
- What models exist for clinical education?
- What are the emerging best practices from across the country?
- What are the facilitators and barriers to clinical education redesign?
- What will be the expected competencies and outcomes of a new model of clinical education?

Within this framework, we identified the emerging themes of both the present and future states to formulate a framework for clinical education redesign.

LITERATURE REVIEW

A keyword search was done using CINAHL and Ovid with the keywords *clinical education, primary care education models, primary care nurse education models, advanced practice nurse clinical education, models of clinical education, innovation in clinical education,* and *inter-professional education.* More than 100 articles were initially retrieved. These were examined at the abstract and title level and retained if the text was written after 2003 and focused on (1) the impact of health care reform on primary care APRN practice or education; (2) the impact of regulations and standards on APRN education; (3) clinical education components for APRNs; (4) the need for innovation or reform in primary care nursing; and (5) interprofessional education models. Articles focusing only on prelicensure education were excluded. A total of 34 articles and reports from the nursing, medical, and allied health literature were the focus of the final review. Most of the literature was descriptive. A topical approach was used to synthesize the themes and patterns found in the overall review.

IMPACT OF PRIMARY CARE APRNS

The primary themes found in the most current literature were focused on the role and positioning of primary care APRNs in health care reform.[3,7,8,15–18] Most of these articles focused on the value and quality of care provided by primary care APRNs. A few included the barriers to effective use of primary care APRNs a result of state-based regulatory issues. Although primary care APRN education was noted as the fastest and least expensive way to address primary care shortages, none of these articles discussed alternative approaches to increase APRN education program capacity.

NURSE PRACTITIONER PREPARATION

Stanley and colleagues[19] described the critical issues faced by nursing programs in expanding APRN education as the need to improve the recruitment and retention of nursing faculty. The limited pool of doctorally prepared faculty and noncompetitive salaries were identified as major barriers to overcoming the diminishing supply of faculty needed for the APRN population to expand. Aiken and colleagues[20] expanded on this discussion to note that new teaching models such as distance learning and simulation will be needed to offset the increasing faculty shortage. They also highlighted the need for increased federal funding support to graduate nursing education as a strategy to increase the supply of both faculty and advanced practice nurses. In the same issue of *Health Affairs*, Cleary and colleagues[21] described the challenges in providing clinical education as another inhibiting factor to the expansion of all nursing education programs. Ridenour[22] stressed that reform is needed in nursing clinical education to focus on team-based clinical education models, interprofessional education, and residencies for APRNs to fully prepare nurses to meet the needs of the future health care system.

In a 2007 study, Hart and Macnee[23] evaluated the perceived preparedness of APRNs for practice after completing their basic nurse practitioner (NP) educational programs. Questionnaires were distributed to a total of 526 attendees at a 2004 NP conference. Only 10% of the respondents perceived that they were very well prepared for practice as an NP after completing their basic NP education. Fifty-one percent perceived they were only somewhat or minimally prepared. No significant differences were noted in age when attending their NP programs, years since graduation, or current age. The authors concluded that formal NP education was not preparing new NPs to feel ready for practice and suggested that more rigorous clinical education needed to be provided by competent experienced NPs who are actively engaged in clinical practice. Barriers to finding appropriate clinical sites and preceptors can include lack of compensation for preceptors, the fear of a negative impact on provider productivity while working with students, and the competition.[24]

Regulatory and accreditation bodies and professional nursing organizations provide guides and standards for nursing programs in developing APRN nursing programs. In 2008, the National League for Nursing sponsored a Think Tank on Transforming Clinical Nursing Education to examine ways to achieve consensus on the structures and processes to transform clinical nursing education. Although primarily focused on prelicensure RN programs, many of the issues and finding were seen as common to all levels of nursing education. Recommendations of this group included the need to effectively support clinical staff who are overburdened with patient care responsibilities as they are asked to participate in educational responsibilities. Education practice partnerships were also noted to be important to new models of clinical education.

CLINICAL EDUCATION REDESIGN

In 2009, the National Organization of Nurse Practitioner Faculties (NONPF) conducted a 4-phase research project funded by the National Council of State Boards of Nursing to clarify information about current and emerging NP educational pathways. Within the 4 phases, the specific aims were (1) identification of the range of NP educational tracks by reviewing Web sites of all schools with master's NP programs; (2) clarification of titling, hours, curriculum, and credentialing information with selected faculty focus groups; (3) validation of information from the focus groups through a survey of all schools with NP educational programs; and (4) prioritization of future directions for NP education. The results of this study quantified the current state of NP educational programs nationally and provided a baseline for implementation of the Consensus Model for APRN Regulation: Licensure, Accreditation, Certification, and Education.[25] Within this study, questions were asked about the components of clinical hours and the use of clinical simulation as direct care hours for NP education. Some of the major findings were that 50.5% of the 295 schools reporting indicated that they used simulation in their NP education and 65.1% counted simulation time as direct care hours. Most of the focus groups expressed interest in moving toward a competency-based approach to NP education. The impact of a competency-based education on credentialing was identified as an area for further clarification. This study provided an evidence base for the development of innovative approaches to NP clinical education redesign.

Stanley and colleagues[19] defined the Consensus Model as the beacon for redesigning APRN education. With acceptance of the Consensus Model, APRN education will become broad based and grounded on 3 separate comprehensive courses of advanced physiology/path physiology, advanced health assessment, and advanced pharmacology as the APRN core. Programs must also prepare graduates with nationally vetted core competencies and must provide sufficient clinical experiences in the role and population focus for certification.

Although several certifying organizations define the number and type of clinical hours required for APRNs to sit for certification examinations, the hours vary from 500 to 600 depending on the NP specialty and organization.[26] This article noted the lack of validation in evidence-based research around the hour requirements. The authors then emphasized that the nursing profession should evaluate the use of technology as a clinical option and other sources including electronic log data to ensure that students are exposed to appropriate amounts and types of clinical experiences and are prepared to provide an efficient and effective foundation for safe practice. Having clinical preceptors more involved with faculty and placement expectations may improve relationships, communication, and the availability of placement opportunities.

In a systematic review of the evidence to enhance student learning in clinical education, DeWolfe and colleagues[27] described the interventions and outcomes of preceptored experiences applicable to health science students. In the set of 47 studies that met the inclusion criteria, the authors identified strategies common to the development of a comprehensive NP preceptor clinical education program. Their findings noted little empiric evidence in the literature about the effectiveness of any particular approach to preceptorship programs but revealed some future directions for the structure, process, and outcomes of clinical education programming. In terms of structure, these authors suggested that preceptors need to be better prepared for their roles through interventions that help them enhance their interactions with students, including assisting students to set goals, developing decision-making skills, and providing effective feedback. In terms of process, the authors found no evidence to recommend individual training and support methods compared with multisession workshops. They recommended the exploration of the use of technology to deliver some areas of clinical education. In discussing outcomes, they focused on the need to develop more conceptual models for practice and research on specific strategies for both preceptors and students. In other studies, several authors have also focused on the potential barriers to precepting NP students and the strategies to recruit, support, and retain preceptors.[28,29] The perceived barriers again included the detrimental effect on productivity of the preceptor, practice not designed to include students, short duration of the precepting experience, discomfort with the teaching roles, and patient expectations for the providers' attention. Preceptor fatigue was also noted as an additional barrier to effective preceptorships.[29] To effectively balance the demands of their work with the time to discuss learning issues with students, preceptors need to know the intrinsic and tangible benefits of being a preceptor and realistic objectives and "just in time" information sharing from faculty during the course of the clinical experience.[28] Although there was little consensus on tangible rewards for preceptors, simple "thank you" notes from students, feedback from faculty, and professional development programs designed to be integrated into the preceptors work schedules were noted as effective strategies for preceptor retention. The key theme that emerged from the discussion of the strategies to improve the clinical experience was the need for partnerships with skilled practitioners, APRN faculty, and NP students.

With the increased focus on the role of primary care APRNs in community health centers, Flinter[30] proposed the concept of formal residency programs in primary care at either the post master's or postdoctoral level as the next step in the evolution of NP preparation. The IOM[1] expanded on this premise to recommend that the Centers for Medicare and Medicaid Services fund the development and implementation of residency programs across all practice settings and evaluate the effectiveness of these programs in expanding competencies and improving patient outcomes. The idea of NP residencies has had a mixed reception, with many arguing that an effective job was done with master's-level preparation. Nonetheless, certain health care centers have begun to implement 1- and 2-year structured, mentored residency experiences for new APRNs, usually at a lesser rate of pay.

Neiderhauser and colleagues[31] encompassed all these perspectives by recommending that nursing programs move from a time-based model of clinical nursing education to a competency-based model and evaluate the evidence to support this type of learning in nursing education. They also suggested that partnerships between nursing education and nursing practice are essential to the development and dissemination of successful innovative models in clinical nursing education. Smith Glasgow and colleagues[32] further broadened this perspective to note that regulations should not be barriers to innovation and that interprofessional models of education are at the core of new clinical education models. They stressed the need to shape the future of health care by creating new models of nursing education and noted that the time for this innovation is now.

INTERPROFESSIONAL MODELS

Derksen and Whelan[9] stressed the need to change the context and content of all health professional education and training models to integrate with health care reform measures. They noted the need to remove the institutional barriers through collaboration among professional organizations, accrediting bodies, and educational institutions to execute meaningful team-based collaborative care and interprofessional education. The disciplines of social work, physical therapy, speech pathology, and pharmacy, osteopathic, chiropractic, and primary care medicine are all in the process of reevaluating and redesigning their clinical education models.[33–38] Each of these disciplines is working to provide clinical education frameworks to enable all health professional students to graduate as competent professionals. Using the IOM[39] model for health professions education as a foundational principle, each discipline is focusing on innovation and collaboration as key components of clinical education models that allow students to develop both the theoretical and practice knowledge, attitudes, and skills to effectively demonstrate competence.

Hodges[40] presented the struggle within medicine to evaluate the competing models of competence development that clearly reflects the issues that are currently being raised within the NP education community. He carefully explored the risks and benefits of a time-based ("tea steeping") model of clinical education in comparison to the newer outcome-based ("i-Doc") model. Although the pure time-based model is described as not being adequate in the current environment of health care, this author suggested that the elements of time should not be completely lost in the development of the outcomes-based approach that is now the focus of health care education redesign.

As noted by the IOM,[1] effective team work among all health care professionals is directly linked to better patient outcomes. Different professional perspectives can be beneficial to patients' well-being. Defined as the occasions "when 2 or more professionals learn with, from and about each other to improve collaboration and the quality of care," interprofessional education has been identified as the most direct approach to enhance the quality of care in health care settings.[41(p.172)] Barnsteiner and colleagues[42] noted that an effective approach to interprofessional learning is common clinical experience, having common patients, projects, and learning objectives. These authors, representing both nursing and medicine, identified the many challenges that must be overcome to design effective interprofessional education models. Included in these challenges are course scheduling, faculty interest and expertise, and the need for agreement on the competencies/capabilities for collaboration across disciplines. Although primarily focused on prelicensure education, this article provided key strategies that can be used across both undergraduate and graduate nursing education as essential components of curriculum focused on the transformation of health care into a safety-critical industry.

In February 2011, a major conference sponsored by the Health Resources and Services Administration, the Josiah Macy Jr Foundation, the Robert Wood Johnson Foundation, and the ABIM Foundation[43] in collaboration with the Inter-professional Education Collaborative was held in Washington, DC. The purpose of this conference was to advance both academic and clinical interprofessional education and to engage all participants in developing a shared vision of the competencies necessary for education and practice. Recognizing the health care workforce shortages and the increased patient demands, particularly in primary care, the conference proceedings described the necessity of increased collaboration and teamwork across the health professions. The conference participants concluded that it is time for a paradigm shift in health professions education and practice. A set of action strategies were identified to support this paradigm shift. These strategies included the need to (1) communicate and disseminate the Inter-professional Education Collaborative core competencies and launch an education campaign that establishes the critical need for interprofessional education and collaboration; (2) develop interprofessional faculty and resources; (3) strengthen metrics and research to identify techniques that work effectively; (4) develop new collaborative academic practices and collaborations with community learning sites; and (5) advance policy changes to support education and research initiatives. The proceeding of this conference served as the precursor for the development of the recently released Core Competencies for Inter-professional Collaborative Practice released in May of 2011.

SUMMARY OF LITERATURE REVIEW

By encompassing literature from a variety of health professions while focusing on NP education and practice, the literature review clearly demonstrates the issues that are affecting the content and context of education across the professions. Health care reform is placing increased demands on all health professions, but with the focus on primary care, APRN education redesign is central to the future of an efficient and effective health care system. The literature review also demonstrates that the most effective approach to clinical education redesign is found in partnerships between education and practice that provide support and effective communication with preceptors. The current dialogue on clinical education redesign is also focused on the change from time-based models to outcome- or competency-based models. Interprofessional education models that incorporate team-based competencies and community education sites seem to be the future vision for the paradigm shift that is being advocated as core to quality, safe health care.

NURSE PRACTITIONER EDUCATION STANDARDS REVIEW

In addition to the themes and trends noted in the literature review, a review of current standards and expectations for NP education provides the additional factors needed to assess the current state of NP education. **Table 1** provides an overview of the standards related to NP clinical education as another element in the gap analysis approach to clinical education redesign.

COMPETENCY REVIEW

The IOM[1] report on health professions education specifies that "all health care professionals should be educated to deliver patient centered care as members of interdisciplinary teams, emphasizing evidence- based practice, quality improvement approaches and informatics" (p. 48). This report has provided the framework for competency-based models across the health professions. The American Academy of Nurse Practitioners[10] recently published a policy brief that focuses on the need for NP students to only progress when they are able to demonstrate and achieve knowledge and competency. The brief stresses that NP education should be competency based, not time based. **Table 2** demonstrates the evolution and commonalties of these competencies across medical and nursing education. Many of the competencies are built on the accrediting standards of the professional organizations.[44,45] With the current discussion of the need for competency/outcome-based models as the foundation of academic and clinical education redesign, this competency comparison provides another foundational element of the gap analysis that serves as the framework for education redesign.

The final element in a review of competency frameworks of APRNs is the definition of competency as defined by the Boards of Registration in Nursing (BORN). For example, the Massachusetts BORN describes competence as "the application of knowledge and the use of affective, cognitive, and psychomotor skills required for the role of a nurse licensed by the Board and for the delivery of safe nursing care in

Table 1
Review of standards related to clinical education of APRN students

Source	Standards
American Association of Colleges of Nursing[49] *The Essentials of Master's Education*	• All graduates of masters programs must have supervised practice experiences that are sufficient to demonstrate mastery of the "essentials." • The term "supervised" is used broadly and can include precepted experiences with faculty site visits. • The development of clinical proficiency is facilitated through the use of focused and sustained clinical experiences designed to strengthen patient care delivery skills and system assessment and interventions skills that will lead to an enhanced understanding of organizational dynamics. • All graduates of a master's nursing program must have supervised clinical experiences that are sufficient to demonstrate mastery of the essentials. • Learning experiences may be accomplished through diverse teaching methodologies including face-to-face and simulated means. • In some instances, the master's student may engage in a clinical experience at the student's employing agency, which may be overseen or supervised by a mentor/preceptor or faculty member. • Sets outcome-focused goals for the clinical learning experiences. • Clinical experiences should be designed as immersion experiences focused on a population or a specific role.

National Organization of Nurse Practitioner Faculties[50] *Clarification of Nurse Practitioner Specialty and Subspecialty Clinical Track Titles, Hours and Credentialing: Report of Four Phased Research Project Conducted by the National Organization of Nurse Practitioner Faculty*	• Phase II of the study focused on clarifying titling, hours, curriculum, and credentialing information in national survey of all schools with master's-level NP programs.
	• Of the 205 respondents, 65.1% indicated that clinical simulation hours should be included in direct clinical hours.
	• Components of clinical hours included.
	   ○ Clinical hours in direct care only.
	   ○ Laboratory and clinical hours are differentiated in various ways.
	   ○ Some skills in laboratory, simulation, or other experiences are included in clinical hours.
	   ○ The range of total clinical clock hours was from 540 to 960.
	• Most participants expressed the need to move toward a competency-based approach to NP education.
	• Suggestions that simulation hours be included as clinical hours.
	• Results noted that although the concepts of outcomes and competencies instead of clinical hours are appealing, it is unclear how certification bodies will react.

(continued on next page)

Table 1
(continued)

Source	Standards

APRN Consensus Work Group and the National Council of State Boards of Nursing APRN Advisory Committee[25]
 	
Consensus Model for APRN Education
	• Ensure clinical and didactic work is comprehensive and sufficient for the graduate to practice in the APRN role and population.
	• Focus on competencies and measurement of competencies.
	• Accreditation by nursing accreditation organization recognized by US Department of Education and/or Council for Higher Education.
	• Incorporates National Council of State Boards Criteria for Evaluating Certification Programs including:
	  ○ Both direct and indirect clinical supervision must be congruent with current national specialty organizations and nursing accreditation guidelines.
	  ○ Supervised clinical experience is directly related to the knowledge and role of the specialty and category.
	Instructional track/major has a minimum of 500 supervised clinical hours overall.

National Task Force on Quality Nurse Practitioner Education[51,52]
 	
Criteria for Evaluation of Practitioner Programs
	• NP faculty members must evaluate students, interface with preceptors, and serve as role models.
	• The didactic and clinical experiences will be sufficient to gain the necessary proficiency in each population focused area.
	• Clinical practice hours refer to hours in which direct clinical care is provided and should be varied and distributed in a way that prepares the student to provide care to the populations served.
	• 500 clinical hours is the minimum that is expected.
	• Adequate faculty, clinical sites and preceptors be available to support the NP clinical education experience
	• NP faculty have the ultimate responsibility for the supervision and evaluation and the oversight of the clinical learning environment.
	  ○ Faculty supervision may be direct or indirect.
	  ○ Direct supervision is when the faculty functions as the on-site preceptor.
	  ○ Indirect supervision has 3 components.
	    ■ Supplementing clinical preceptor teaching
	    ■ Acting as liaison with the agency
	    ■ Evaluating student's progress
	  ○ The recommended on-site faculty-student ratio is 1:2 if faculty are not seeing patients and 1:1 if faculty are seeing patients.
	  ○ The ratio for indirect supervision is 1:6.

- Each nursing program should document how they assign faculty: based on defined faculty workload or amount of designated faculty time.
  - Ratios may vary relative to certain practice areas and the individual faculty member.
- The intent of the faculty-student ratio is based on the premise that the preparation of competent health care providers is a faculty intense process that requires faculty role modeling and direct student evaluation to determine competence.
- The ratio should take into account the cumulative teaching/administrative duties of the faculty member and his or her clinical practice.
- Faculty may share the clinical teaching with qualified preceptors.
- Preceptors should have preparation and at least 1 year of clinical experience in their areas of clinical education.
- The competence of preceptors and faculty should be evaluated annually.
- Future considerations discussed the possible need to increase clinical time.

American Association of Colleges of Nursing[53]
The Essential Clinical Resources for Nursing's Academic Mission

- Students are best served by opportunities to work together and learn with nurse mentors, preceptors, and role models.
- Clinical site–based learning for graduate nurse education requires a sufficient number of educationally and experientially qualified practitioners who are willing and competent to serve as preceptors and role models.
- Graduate students provide direct care in the advance practice role to a suitable number of patients whose health problems/needs are sufficiently representative to prepare them for professional practice in the area in which they are being prepared.
- Nursing education leaders promote reexamination of traditional models/approaches to clinical education to include:
  - Redefinition of education/service partnerships to promote cohesion between faculty and clinicians
  - Recognition of the worth and contribution of clinical staff to the educational mission of nursing education
  - Increase in faculty participation in the clinical arena
  - Fostering of innovative and collaborative partnerships with a variety of health and social service institutions
  - Nursing leaders encourage and support faculty practice in all of its forms
  - Educators examine the nursing education culture, including reward systems, with respect to relationships, partnerships, and reconnections with nursing practice.
- Recommend that nursing education leaders promote reexamination of traditional models/approaches to clinical nursing education.
- Provides listing of nursing programs across country with innovative models.

Table 2
Competency review

Source	Competencies
IOM[39] Health Professions Education: A Bridge to Quality, *Competencies for All Health Care Professionals*	All health professionals should be educated to deliver patient-centered care as members of an interdisciplinary team, emphasizing evidence-based practice, quality improvement approaches, and informatics.
Accrediting Council for Graduate Medical Education[44]: *ACGME Outcome Project*	• Practice-based learning and improvement • Systems-based practice • Patient care • Interpersonal and communication skills • Professionalism • Medical knowledge

QSEN,[45] *Quality and Safety Education for Advanced Nursing Practice*	These competencies build on the earlier prelicensure competencies with the knowledge, attitudes and skills (KSAs) specific to APRN practice and are proposed to stimulate development of teaching strategies in programs preparing the next generation of APRNs.
	  • Patient-centered care
	  • Teamwork and collaboration
	  • Evidence-based practice
	  • Quality improvement
	  • Safety
	  • Informatics

Department of Higher Education Nursing Initiative,[54] *Nurse of the Future Core Nursing Competencies*	Definitions of the competencies are for all nurses. KSAs for prelicensure:
	  • Patient-centered care
	  • Professionalism
	  • Leadership
	  • Systems-based practice
	  • Informatics and technology
	  • Communication
	  • Teamwork and collaboration
	  • Safety
	  • Quality improvement
	  • Evidence-based practice

American Academy of Nurse Practitioners and National Organization of Nurse Practitioner Faculty[55] *Domains and Competencies of Nurse Practitioner Practice*	Content domains (with specific competencies/actions within each domain)
	  • Management of patient health/illness
	  • The nurse practitioner–patient relationship
	  • The teaching-coaching function
	  • Professional role
	  • Managing and negotiating health care systems
	  • Monitoring and ensuring the quality of health care practices
	  • Culturally sensitive care

(*continued on next page*)

Table 2
(continued)

Source	Competencies
The Hartford Institute for Geriatric Nursing and the National Organization of Nurse Practitioner Faculties,[56] *Adult-Gerontology Primary Care Nurse Practitioner Competencies*	Competency document contains a side-by-side comparison with National Organization of Nurse Practitioner Faculties (NONPF) domains and competencies. Each general competency area has a competency statement with detailed competencies/actions listed under each that are more specific than NONPF domains <ul><li>Health promotion, health protection, disease prevention and treatment</li><li>Nurse practitioner–patient relationship</li><li>Teaching-coaching function</li><li>Professional role</li><li>Managing and negotiating health care delivery systems</li><li>Monitoring and ensuring the quality of health care practice</li><li>Cultural and spiritual competence</li></ul>
National Organization of Nurse Practitioner Faculties (2011),[52] *Nurse Practitioner Core Competencies*	Competency document emphasizes the independent and interprofessional practice and the analytic skills for evaluating and providing evidence-based, patient-centered care across settings and are consistent with the IOM[1] report. Each general competency area has a listing of more specific competencies/actions. <ul><li>Scientific foundation competencies</li><li>Leadership competencies</li><li>Quality competencies</li><li>Practice inquiry competencies</li><li>Technology and information literacy competencies</li><li>Policy competencies</li><li>Health delivery systems competencies</li><li>Ethics competencies</li><li>Independent practice competencies</li></ul>
American Association of Colleges of Nursing, American Association of Colleges of Osteopathic Medicine, Association of Schools of Public Health, American Association of Colleges of Colleges of Pharmacy, American Dental Education Association, American Association of Medical Colleges,[57] *Core Competencies for Inter-professional Collaborative Practice*	Competencies were formulated to be translated into learning objectives; are general in nature to function as guidelines; generally focused on prelicensure and precertification levels. Encourage education–practice links and how as well of what type of care is delivered. Document contains graphic representations of interprofessionality, framework for action on interprofessional education, and collaborative practice and approaches to transforming education. Each competency domain has a general competency statement with specific roles/ responsibilities competencies. <ul><li>Competency domain 1: Values/ethics for professional practice</li><li>Competency domain 2: Roles and responsibilities</li><li>Competency domain 3: Interprofessional communication</li><li>Competency domain 4: Teams and teamwork</li></ul>

accordance with accepted standards of practice."[46] The BORN further notes that (1) competency includes only those areas of practice for which the APRN has formal, advanced nursing education and documented competency; (2) certification is one measure of competence; and (3) additional education through experience and continuing education is another measure of competence. The process of using competencies to frame curriculum redesign involves the review and development of learning objectives and learning activities and the identification of the factors that influence the choice of learning activities.[43] In addition, a competency-based framework can generate the ideas for faculty to transform their curriculum, teaching strategies, and clinical experiences to meet the demands of the redesigned health care system.[45]

SUMMARY

Dentzer[47] noted that no one should underestimate the magnitude of the changes that will have to be made in education, regulations, and practice as health care reform reinvents primary care. The traditional models of education for nurses and all health care professionals are in the middle of radical transformation in response to the rapidly changing health care environment.[2] Breakthrough ideas and innovation will emerge as nurse educators respond to these challenges. In his work, *Change by Design*, Tim Brown[48] described the design-thinking process that is necessary for creative problem solving. When small teams of talented, optimisticm and collaborative thinkers come together, the creative process begins with discovering what constraints exist and establishing a framework to evaluate them. The overlapping criteria for success in innovation are feasibility (what is possible in the foreseeable future), viability (what is likely to become part of a sustainable model), and desirability (what makes sense and has value). This process combined with an emphasis on fundamental human needs is what drives design thinking.[48]

This design-thinking process can be applied to a variety of settings and may provide the opportunity to turn APRN clinical education redesign into tangible outcomes. APRN educators across the country are working in small motivated groups to create new models that can meet the challenges facing APRN education and practice. The gap analysis process contained in this report provides a detailed look at the feasibility, viability, and desirability components of design thinking. The detailed literature, standards, and competency reviews and the update on the interprofessional models now emerging provide an overview of current expectations and insight into future opportunities for APRN education redesign. Armed with this information, creative faculty, in concert with practice partners, should be fully prepared to bridge the gap between thinking and doing, unleash their design thinking, and create the innovation needed in APRN clinical education.

REFERENCES

1. Institute of Medicine. The future of nursing: leading change, advancing health. Washington, DC: National Academies Press; 2010.
2. Benner P, Sutphen M, Leonard V, et al. Educating nurses: a call for radical reform. San Francisco (CA): Jossey-Bass; 2010.
3. Koeniger-Donahue R, Hawkins J. The future of nursing and health care: through the looking glass 2030. J Am Acad Nurse Pract 2010;22:233–5.
4. Starfield BL, Shi L, Macinko J. Contribution of primary care to health systems and health. Milbank Q 2005;83(3):457–502.

5. Creating jobs and increasing the number of primary care providers: fact sheet. 2010. Available at: http://www.Healthcare.gov/news/factsheets. Accessed February 16, 2011.
6. O'Neill Hewlett P, Bleich M. The reemergence of academic-service partnerships: responses to the nursing shortage, work environment issues, and beyond. J Prof Nurs 2004;23(5):273–4.
7. Naylor M, Kurtzman E. The role of nurse practitioners in reinventing primary care. Health Aff 2010;29(5):893–9.
8. Bodenheimer T, Hoangmai HP. Primary care: current problems and proposes solutions. Health Aff 2010;29(5):799–805.
9. Derksen D, Whelan E. Closing the health care workforce gap: Reforming federal workforce policies to meet the needs of the 21st century. Center for American Progress. 2009. Available at: http://www.americanprogress.org/issues/2010/01/health_workforce.html. Accessed February 14, 2011.
10. American Academy of Nurse Practitioners. Clinical outcomes: The yardstick of educational effectiveness. 2011. Available at: http://aanp.org/NR/rdonlyres/B0A76B9B-4EDC-46F6-A35CFD5AEF68020E/4711/ClinicalOutcomesTheYardstickofEducational Effective.pdf. Accessed January 21, 2011.
11. American Academy of Nurse Practitioners. Nurse practitioners in primary care. 2011. Available at: http://aanp.org/NR/rdonlyres/9AF1A29F-5C82-4151-98CB-22D1F20A9BD9/0/NPsInPrimaryCare324.pdf. Accessed January 21, 2011.
12. American Academy of Nurse Practitioners. Position statement on nurse practitioner curriculum. 2010. Available at: http://aanp.org/NR/rdonlyres/59523729-0179-466A-A7FB-BDEE68160E8E/0/2010Curriculum.pdf. Accessed January 21, 2011.
13. Business Dictionary. Gap analysis. 2011. Available at: http://www.businessdictionary.com/definition/gap-analysis.html. Accessed November 9, 2010.
14. Charles A. Dana Center. Gap analysis. 2004. Available at: www.utdanacenter.org/downloads/presentations/gapanalysis_March04pdf. Accessed November 9, 2010.
15. Buerhaus P. Have nurse practitioners reached a tipping point: interview of a panel of NP thought leaders. Nurs Econ 2010;28(5):346–9.
16. Clark Graham M. New era of health care affords new opportunities. Nurse Pract 2010;35(7):15.
17. Fairman J, Rowe J, Hasmiller S, et al. Broadening the scope of nursing practice. N Engl J Nursing 2011;364(3):193–6.
18. Aiken L. Nurses for the future. N Engl J Med 2011. Available at: www.nejm.org.
19. Stanley J, Werner K, Apple K. Positioning advanced practice registered nurses for health care reform: consensus on APRN regulation. J Prof Nurs 2009;25(6):340–8.
20. Aiken L, Cheung R, Olds D. Education policy initiatives to address the nurse shortage in the United States. Health Aff 2009;28(4):w646–56.
21. Cleary B, Mcbride BA, McClure M, et al. Expanding the capacity of nursing education. Health Affairs 2009;2(4):w634–45. http://dx.doi.org/10.1377/hithaff.28.4.w634.
22. Ridenour N. Clinical education reform: reenvisioning the workforce. J Nurs Educ 2009;48(8):419–20.
23. Hart A, Macnee C. How well are nurse practitioners prepared for practice: Results of a 2004 questionnaire study. J Am Acad Nurse Pract 2007;19:35–42.
24. Brooks MV, Niederhauser VP. Preceptor expectations and issues with nurse practitioner clinical rotations. J Am Acad Nurse Pract 2010;22:573–9.
25. APRN Consensus Work Group, the National Council of State Boards of Nursing APRN Advisory Council. Consensus model for APRN regulation: licensure, accreditation, certification & education. 2008. Available at: http://nonpf.

com/associations/10789/files/APRNConsensusmodelfinal.pdf. Accessed December 7, 2011.

26. Bray C, Koozer Olson K. Family nurse practitioner clinical requirements: Is the best recommendation 500 hours? J Am Acad Nurse Pract 2009;21:135–9.

27. De Wolfe J, Perkin C, Harrison M, et al. Strategies to prepare and support preceptors and students for preceptorship: a systematic review. Nurse Educ 2010;35(3):98–100.

28. DeWolfe JA, Laschinger S, Perkin C. Preceptors' perspective on recruitment, support, and retention of preceptors. J Nurs Educ 2010;49(4):198–206.

29. Barker E, Pitmann O. Becoming a super preceptor: A practical guide to preceptorship in today's clinical climate. J Am Acad Nurse Pract 2010;22:144–9.

30. Flinter M. Residency programs for primary care nurse practitioners in federally qualified health centers: a service perspective. Online J Issues Nurs 2005; 10(3). http://dx.doi.org/10.3912/OJIN.Vol10No03Man05.

31. Neiderhauser V, MacIntyre R, Garner C, et al. Transformational partnerships in nursing education. Nurs Educ Perspect 2010;31(6):353–5.

32. Smith Glasgow M, Dunphy L, Mainous R. Innovative nursing educational curriculum for the 21st century. Nurs Educ Perspect 2010;31(6):353–7.

33. Hayhurst C. Learning together: inter-professional education programs. PT in Motion 2010;2(3):22–7.

34. Meyers F, Weinberger S, Fitzgibbons J, et al. Redesigning residency training in internal medicine: the consensus report of the Alliance for Academic Internal Medicine Education Redesign Taskforce. Acad Med 2007;82(12):1211–8.

35. Frey A, Dupper D. A broader conceptual approach to clinical practice for the 21st century. Child Schools 2005;17(1):33–44.

36. Riva J, Lam J, Stanford E, et al. Inter-professional education through shadowing experiences in multi-disciplinary clinical settings. Chiropr Osteopat 2010;18. http://dx.doi.org/10.1186/1746-1340-18-31.

37. Stanfield J. Issues and innovation in clinical education: Regulation, collaboration and communication. Adv Speech Lang Pathol 2005;7(3):173–6.

38. Wetherbee E, Peatman N, Kenney D, et al. Standards for clinical education: a qualitative study. J Phys Ther Educ 2010;24(3):35–43.

39. Institute of Medicine. Health professions education; A bridge to quality. Washington, DC: Author; 2003.

40. Hodges B. A tea-steeping or i-doc model for medical education. Acad Med 2010; 85(9):s34–44.

41. Silver I, Leslie K. Faculty development for continuing interprofessional education and collaborative practice. J Contin Educ Health 2009;29(3):172–7. http://dx.doi.org/10.1002/chp.20032.

42. Barnsteiner J, Disch J, Hall L, et al. Promoting inter-professional education. Nurs Outlook 2007;55:144–50.

43. Josiah Macy Jr. Foundation, Robert Wood Johnson Foundation, ABIM Foundation, IPEC Collaborative Conference proceedings. Team-based competencies; Building a shared foundation for education and clinical practice. 2011. Available at: http://www.aamc.org/download1186752/data/teambased_competencies pdf.

44. Accreditation Council for Graduate Medical Education. ACGME outcome project. 2006. Available at: http://www.ACGME.org/outcome/comp/compfullasp. Accessed January 7, 2010.

45. Cronenwett L, Sherwood G, Pohl J, et al. Quality and safety education for advanced nursing practice. Nurs Outlook 2009;57:338–48. http://dx.doi.org/10.1016/joutlook.2009.07.009.

46. Massachusetts Board of Registration in Nursing–BORN. Preparing for advanced practice nursing. 2011. Available at: http://www.mass.gov/Eeohhs2/docs/dph/regs/244cmr009.pdf. Accessed January 11, 2011.

47. Dentzer S. Reinventing primary care: a task that is far "too important to fail". Health Aff 2011;29(5):757.

48. Brown T. Change by design. New York: HarperCollins; 2009.

49. American Association of Colleges of Nursing. The essentials of master's education. Washington, DC: Author; 2011.

50. National Organization of Nurse Practitioner Faculties. Clarification of nurse practitioner specialty and subspecialty clinical track titles, hours and credentialing: Report of four-phased research project conducted by the National Organization of Nurse Practitioner Faculties. 2009. Available at: http://nonpf.com/associations/10789/files/projectfinal report.pdf. Accessed February 9, 2010.

51. National Task Force on Quality Nurse Practitioner Education. Criteria for evaluation of nurse practitioner programs. Washington, DC: Author; 2012.

52. National Organization of Nurse Practitioner Faculties. Nurse practitioner core competencies. 2011. Available at: http://nonpf.com/associations/10789/files/IntegratedNPcorecompetencies/FinalApril2011.pdf. Accessed June 10, 2011.

53. American Association of Colleges of Nursing. The essential clinical resources for nursing's academic mission. 2007. Available at: http://nonpf.com/associations/10789files/NTFevalcriteria2008finalpdf. Accessed May 4, 2011.

54. Massachusetts Department of Higher Education Nurse of the Future Competency Committee. Nurse of the future nursing core competencies. Boston: Author; 2010.

55. National Organization of Nurse Practitioner Faculties. Domains and core competencies of nurse practitioner practice. 2006. Available at: http://nonpf.com/displaycommon.cfm?an=1&subarticlenbr=14. Accessed May 8, 2010.

56. American Association of Colleges of Nursing, The Hartford Institute for Geriatric Nursing at New York University, National Organization of Nurse Practitioner Faculties. Adult-gerontology primary care nurse practitioner competencies. 2010. Available at: http://www.aacn.nche.edu/Education/curriculum/adultgeroprimcareNPcomp.pdf. Accessed January 9, 2011.

57. American Association of Colleges of Nursing, American Association of Colleges of Osteopathic Medicine, American Association of Colleges of Pharmacy, American Dental Education Association, Association of American Medical Colleges, Association of Schools of Public Health. Core competencies for inter-professional collaborative practice. 2011. Available at: www.aacn.nche.edu/Education/pdf/IPECReport.pdf. Accessed December 5, 2011.

Testing Computer-Based Simulation to Enhance Clinical Judgment Skills in Senior Nursing Students

Deborah L. Weatherspoon, PhD(c), CRNA, RN[a],*,
Tami H. Wyatt, PhD, RN, CNE[b]

KEYWORDS

- Experiential learning theory • Nursing education • Simulation
- Computer-based simulation • Clinical judgment

KEY POINTS

- In nursing education, experiential learning is augmented through the use of simulated clinical experiences provided in simulation laboratories.
- A variety of simulations have been reported; however, few studies target the effectiveness of experiential learning through the use of a computer-based simulation available to the individual user.
- An educational intervention based on Kolb's Experiential Learning Theory (ELT) is examined in this pilot study to determine the feasibility of conducting a future larger-scale research project on the effectiveness of ELT to enhance the development of clinical judgment skills.

SIMULATION ENHANCING CLINICAL JUDGMENT

The professional nurse must engage in complex cognition to critically examine multiple variables and make clinical judgments that promote patient care. Reflection about the care of a patient, in the context of the situation, is the basis for judgment.[1–3] The judgment, when used to determine a nursing intervention, exemplifies theoretical science, or the application of knowledge, with practical experience regarding patient care.[4,5] Expert clinical practice requires a nurse to quickly and efficiently evaluate a patient's condition including observed data, and determine an immediate intervention to achieve desired patient outcomes.[5,6]

[a] School of Nursing, Middle Tennessee State University, 1603 Wellington Court, Murfreesboro, TN 37066, USA; [b] HITS Lab, Education Technology & Simulation, College of Nursing, University of Tennessee Knoxville, 1200 Volunteer Boulevard, Knoxville, TN 37996-4180, USA
* Corresponding author.
E-mail addresses: Deborah.Weatherspoon@mtsu.edu; dweatherspoon56@gmail.com

Nurs Clin N Am 47 (2012) 481–491
http://dx.doi.org/10.1016/j.cnur.2012.07.002
0029-6465/12/$ – see front matter © 2012 Elsevier Inc. All rights reserved.

The result of poor clinical judgment may lead to detrimental patient outcomes exemplified by "failure to rescue" behavior.[7] An example is found in high-risk areas, such as triage nursing in the emergency department, where patient acuity must be accurately and efficiently determined. Assigning too high of an acuity level may result in the delay of treatment of another patient with a more serious condition, while assigning an acuity level that is too low may lead to a poor outcome for the presenting patient. Nurses clearly must make clinical judgments while providing care and, therefore, student nurses must learn the techniques that require complex cognition. However, in the increasingly complex clinical environment, and especially in high-acuity areas of care, many students and new graduates lack the needed skills for expert clinical judgment.[8] This elusive skill set requires both cognitive gain and experience,[9,10] and teaching the critical thinking skills of clinical judgment may be a challenge for nurse educators.

Most research conducted on educational methods for improving clinical judgment has focused on deliberative and analytical application of scientific knowledge. In the complex world of nursing, expert clinical judgment exceeds the deliberate, conscious, decision-making characteristic of competent performance to include the holistic and intuitive response gained through experiential learning.[11] Benner[12] described 5 levels of nursing expertise in her sentinel work *From Novice to Expert*. Using a model that focuses on actual performance and outcomes in specific situations, the levels of expertise are defined not only by nurses' knowledge but also by their perceptual acuity. Benner posits that clinical judgment is gained through experiential learning that includes reflections on past concrete experiences.[11] In nursing education experiential learning occurs in a skills laboratory and in actual, often limited, clinical encounters with patients.[13] Innovative educational strategies aimed at developing clinical judgment skills prepare the prelicensure professional nurse for quality patient care and fewer failure-to-rescue behaviors. Simulation laboratories have gained great acceptance in education as a strategy to enhance clinical judgment through experiential learning. However, research grounded in a strong theoretical base is needed to design and support effective strategies to meet this goal. An educational intervention based on Kolb's Experiential Learning Theory (ELT)[14] is examined in this pilot study to determine the feasibility of conducting a future larger-scale research project on the effectiveness of ELT to enhance the development of clinical judgment skills.

SIMULATION AND KOLB'S EXPERIENTIAL LEARNING THEORY

Kolb asserts that "Learning, the creation of knowledge and meaning, occurs through the active extension and grounding of ideas and experiences in the external world and through internal reflection about the attributes of these experiences and ideas."[14(p52)] Kolb's ELT was based on this definition and the work of others scholars' theories that include experience as a central role. According to ELT, learning occurs through two dialectically opposed adaptive orientations that guide the comprehension of information.[14] ELT defines a process that follows a cyclical arrangement of an Act, or concrete experience; Reflection on the experience; Conceptualization of the experience; and Experimentation (action or decision making). This active process is applied in real or simulated experiences.[14]

Simulations are defined as the artificial replication of real-world situations designed to provide a safe and nonthreatening, interactive learning environment in which students can practice clinical scenarios, psychomotor skills, and develop critical thinking skills.[15–17] The use of simulation is not new to nursing, and has been used successfully for more than 20 years in a variety of methods and settings. Simulation offers a rich environment to operationalize and test ELT's effectiveness for enhancing clinical judgment.

Simulated clinical experiences typically begin with a clinical picture, or case scenario; this initial event is what Kolb terms direct apprehension of a concrete experience. This scenario is followed by transformation of the experience through self-reflection, and includes opposing dialectical thoughts that weigh what is currently experienced (seen, heard, touched) and what is known about similar situations from past experience, intuition, and cognitive knowledge. Having reflected on the experience, abstract comprehension occurs when the learner makes sense of the occurrence and forms a logical basis for decision making and clinical judgment. Finally a clinical judgment is made, which correlates to extension or active experimentation; according to ELT, this step transforms the abstract comprehension by testing it in practice. During the simulation, a clinical judgment in the form of a decision leads the person back to another concrete experience (what happened based on their decision).

LITERATURE ON SIMULATION AND CLINICAL JUDGMENT

Simulation is considered any mock clinical situation, and the delivery of simulation may range from low-technology case studies to high-fidelity, realistic, and sophisticated patient simulators.[18] A mainstay and perhaps a pioneer in experiential learning is the traditional paper case study. The use of case studies in education has been documented for more than 100 years; the typical use is to apply theories and didactic content to simulations of potential real-life events.[19] Case studies may be in-depth descriptions of the scenario or be more detailed, focusing on a specific problem. DeYoung[20] asserts the use of case study allows learners to apply their previous experiences to new learning. Several scholars assert that case-study learning improves problem solving, decision making, critical thinking, and self-directed learning.[19,21] Earlier studies support that the use of case studies for problem-based study increased enthusiasm and motivation in nursing.[22]

Much of the literature on simulation in nursing education has focused on instructor-led simulations, particularly with the explosion of high-fidelity patient simulation. The cost of high-fidelity patient simulators requires substantial time and a financial commitment. Although recommended sessions should be short, the group size is typically small, with assigned role play.[8] An adequate number of educators are required to facilitate the actual simulation and conduct debriefing. Managing large classes of nursing students may require several days and allow only one attempt by each student. Because of these constraints, educators may continue to rely on low-fidelity simulation, such as case studies, to augment experiential learning. Although paper case studies offer a patient scenario and many offer feedback with correct answers, they may not fit the high-tech learning style of today's typical nursing student. An alternative may be a computer-based simulation that incorporates patient scenarios similar to paper case studies, in an interactive gaming-style format.

Computer-based simulation is a computer screen–based program designed for an individual player that includes many aspects of computer-based gaming. Games provide a risk-free space to apply learned knowledge in a virtual environment. Werth and Werth[23] describe gaming as educational strategies that include delivering small chunks of information with interactive trial-and-error activities that allow risk-taking in a safe environment. Computer-based simulation offers a continuous feed of problems, or descriptive case studies, and the player determines a course of action followed by feedback. A scoring method may be available with an option to compete with other players in the virtual world. This type of learning offers independence, self direction, and applicability of learned knowledge in a context that is familiar to today's learner. Computer-based simulation games are interactive, challenging, and give feedback without requiring the educator to invest additional time and resources in creating the feedback.[24]

In a virtual-reality learning environment, educators may provide experiential learning opportunities that through active participation facilitate problem solving and clinical judgment on the patient's care.[25–27] The use of computer-based simulation as an educational resource may facilitate student nurses' ability to provide evidence-based nursing care while reflecting, synthesizing, and applying knowledge in various contexts, rather than a competence-based role. In addition, the simulated environment allows students an opportunity to choose priority nursing interventions with immediate feedback of patient outcomes in a safe learning environment. Computer-based simulation is convenient because it resides on any computer, availability being restricted only by the limitations of access to the computer. Programs that provide instant feedback support the needs of today's learners for guidance that supports reflection and enhances critical thinking skills.

At present, there is no literature published on how computer-based simulation affects clinical judgment and critical thinking skills in the prelicensure student nurse. The research question in the research reported here was: Would a computer-based simulation game improve a student's clinical judgment? The overall aim of this pilot study was to determine the feasibility of using a computer-based simulation with senior nursing students to improve clinical judgment. It is believed that the use of computer-based simulation, when compared with standard printed case-study scenarios, will increase students' clinical judgment as demonstrated by their accuracy and efficiency in prioritizing the necessities of patient care.

METHODS

This study used a pretest-intervention-posttest experimental design with a randomly selected control and experimental group to determine the feasibility of a computer-based simulation in improving student's clinical judgment. Once the study was approved by the Institutional Review Board, the participants were recruited from baccalaureate nursing programs who were seniors, enrolled in a local university in the Southeast, and older than 18 years. The population recruited for this study was primarily female, with approximately 5% to 10% being male. The majority of students were non–degree-holding students with a median age of 22 years. All had completed their general education courses and were enrolled full-time in nursing courses that included clinical experiences. All senior nursing students in their final semester before graduation were invited to participate. Thirty-two participants were recruited and 23 participants voluntarily enrolled in the study. Following initial recruitment, written consent was obtained from all participants. None of the participants withdrew once the study began.

Intervention

A computer simulation was sought that targeted advanced clinical judgment skills for nurses. Clinical areas with potentially high acuity and a rapid pace were considered. Emergency triage was selected because of the high levels of clinical judgment necessary in this nursing role. Triage is a system to rank patients according to the severity of their condition and their need for medical care, irrespective of the order of arrival or other factors such as age, ethnicity, or religion.[28] Triage is an inherently complex and dynamic process that requires rapid assessment and prioritization of patients, often with limited information.[29] Failure to recognize and prioritize those who have the most urgent problems and are in need of immediate care may lead to serious negative outcomes, including death.[30] However, the overcautious triage nurse may jeopardize other patients by increasing their wait times when a high-priority level is assigned to a patient unnecessarily. Typically the role of triage nurse is assigned to the most experienced nurses; however, this notion is being challenged and more nurses with limited experience are filling the role. Considine and colleagues[31] found that specific educational preparation and appropriate decision support tools enable less experienced nurses to work effectively in emergency triage. For these reasons described, emergency triage was considered a good fit for innovative teaching strategies that increase knowledge and experience in a safe environment with the goal of increasing clinical judgment.

A product offered by SwiftRiver Online Learning titled Emergency Room Triage Software[32] was used for the experiential education intervention. The simulation included short descriptive case studies that required the user to assign an acuity level, an emergency room (there are choices of standard rooms or trauma rooms), and an appropriately trained nurse (higher acuity levels require a more experienced nurse than lower acuity levels). The simulation prompted players with messages, for example, "You failed to admit a higher acuity patient first." The simulation did not have an unfolding scenario; it was static in the presentation of options so that each student had the same experience. A screenshot of the game is shown in **Fig. 1.**

Instrument

The instrument was developed by the researcher for this study and is known as the Triage Acuity Instrument (TAI). The TAI was based on the *Emergency Severity Index, Version 4: Implementation Handbook* (Gilboy and colleagues, 2005) and consists of multiple short case presentations representing a patient presenting to the Emergency Department. The instrument is designed to test the clinical judgment skills by measuring the user's ability to accurately assign patient acuity scores as defined by

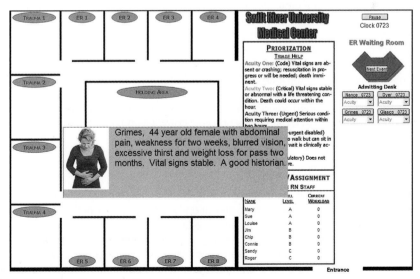

Fig. 1. SwiftRiver Emergency Room Simulator.

the Emergency Severity Index.[33] The score was based on the total number of questions answered correctly in the allotted time.

Before the study, the TAI was reviewed for validity by 2 experienced nurse educators with expertise in test and measurements. Both agreed that TAI assessment results should satisfy the validity criteria listed by Nitko[34]; in particular, content representativeness and relevance; representation of thinking skills and processes; reliability and objectivity; fairness to different types of students; and economy, efficiency, practicality, and instructional features.

Procedures

The study began with a standardized lecture on triage to all participants given by a course instructor, who was not a part of this research team. Following the lecture all participants completed the TAI as the pretest. The test was administered in a quiet, comfortable classroom, and demographic information forms were completed. The TAI was designed to test for accuracy and efficiency. Accuracy was assessed as the total number of correct responses and efficiency was determined as the number of correct responses within a time limit of 30 minutes. The instrument contained more questions than could be answered within the time limit. The purpose was to provide a method to test for the maximum number of answers in a finite period of time as a correlation of efficiency.

Following completion of the pretest, one half of the students were randomly assigned to the experimental (A) group and half to the control (B) group. The control group remained in the classroom and the experimental group was relocated to the computer laboratory.

After a 15-minute break, Group A was instructed to begin the intervention of the single-player simulated computer game. The simulation began with a basic description of how to play. During the same time period the control group participants remained in the classroom and received a paper study guide. The study guide was compiled using the case studies supplied by the simulation developer; therefore, it covered the same scenarios used in the simulation intervention. Nurse educators commonly use the case-study approach to augment teaching.[35] The case study may briefly describe a typical client with a disorder, treatment, or situation, and ask the student to explain the connection between symptoms and signs or to determine a nursing intervention.[35] During the intervention time, no further instructions were given to either the control or the experimental groups. The participants worked individually for a period of 1 hour.

Immediately following the intervention and a 15-minute break, the participants were given the TAI as a posttest. As previously described, a 30-minute time limit was maintained and testing stopped when time was called. After completion of the posttest, the researcher announced that data collection was complete and thanked the subjects for their participation.

DATA ANALYSES AND RESULTS

Before attempting statistical analyses of test data, an informal evaluation of the dependent variable (posttest score) distribution for both the control and experimental groups was performed using box plots and Q-Q plots. No serious threats to normality were noted. Because this was a pilot study, pretest scores for both groups, overall (control plus experimental groups) pretest scores, and overall (pretest plus posttest) scores were also evaluated using box plots and Q-Q plots. Again, no serious threats to normality were noted; however, the pretest scores for the experimental group reflected a skewed-right distribution. In attempting to determine the effects of control-experimental group interventions, analyses focused on differences between pretest and posttest performance and the influence of sample demographic variables. Because of the large observed difference between control group and experimental group pretest scores (**Table 1**), study variables were analyzed using repeated-measures analysis of variance (ANOVA) and t-tests, both independent-sample and paired-sample. A repeated-measures ANOVA was performed to investigate interaction of time (from pretest to posttest) by group and to determine if there was a change in test scores over time. The Levene test of equality of error variances was not significant for either pretest or posttest. The interaction of time by group was not significant, $F(1,21) = 3.863$, $P = .063$, partial $\eta^2 = .155$, indicating that scores of both groups changed similar amounts from pretest to posttest. The main effect of time was significant, $F(1,21) = 34.007$, $P<.001$, partial $\eta^2 = .618$, pointing to a global change in test scores from pretest to posttest. While most subjects in each of the study groups experienced an increase in number of correct responses from pretest to posttest, one subject in both the control and experimental groups scored lower on the posttest than on the pretest.

Because the pretest means for the control group (mean = 74.273, 95% confidence interval [CI] 63.231–85.315) and the experimental group (mean = 56.250, 95% CI 45.678–66.822) were so far apart, independent t-tests were run to determine if the groups differed in pretest scores, age, or experience. (There was insufficient variability for testing differences in education, race, or gender.) As expected, a Levene test for equality of variances indicated that the variance of the pretest scores for the control and experimental groups was significant, $t(21) = 2.45$, $P = .023$. No significant differences were found in age, $t(21) = .073$, $P = .943$, or experience, $t(21) = 1.96$, $P = .068$.

Again, because the control and experimental groups differed so greatly in pretest means, comparing the degree of improvement between them was difficult. Thus, paired t-tests were run for each group to compare pretest and posttest scores. The control group pretest-posttest mean difference was −20.000 (standard deviation [SD] = 21.029) correct responses, whereas the experimental group pretest-posttest mean difference was −40.333 (SD = 27.763) correct responses. The experimental group showed a very significant improvement, $t(11) = -5.033$, $P<.001$; the control group showed a marginally significant improvement, $t(10) = -3.154$, $P = .010$. The effect size was large, with Cohen's $d = .97$.

Assessment score reliability, pretest and posttest, was indicated by means, standard error of means, and 95% CI for groups, time, and groups by time (**Table 2**). It should be observed, however, that the comparatively low pretest score mean of the experimental group and its skewed-right distribution may not be representative of

Table 1
Group statistics for test performance, age, and experience

	Group	N	Mean	Std. Deviation	Std. Error Mean
Pre-test Score (# correct)	Control	11	74.27	19.432	5.859
	Experiment	12	56.25	15.772	4.553
Post-test Score (# correct)	Control	11	94.27	20.180	6.084
	Experiment	12	96.58	32.250	9.310
Age (years)	Control	11	24.91	6.332	1.909
	Experiment	12	25.08	5.178	1.495
Experience (months)	Control	11	17.64	20.432	6.160
	Experiment	12	4.08	10.698	3.088

Table 2
Overall means for group test scores, time (Pre-and Post-Test), and groups x time

Factor	Group or Test	Mean	Std. Error	95% Confidence Interval Lower Bound	Upper Bound
Group	Control	84.273	5.806	72.198	96.347
	Experimental	76.417	5.559	64.856	87.977
Time	Pre-Test	65.261	3.675	57.618	72.905
	Post-Test	95.428	5.673	83.631	107.225
Groups x time	Control Pre-test	74.273	5.310	62.231	85.315
	Control Post-test	94.273	8.195	77.231	111.315
	Experimental Pre-test	56.250	5.084	45.678	66.822
	Experimental Post-test	96.583	7.846	80.267	112.900

future samples from the population under study. Still, the small magnitudes of the standard errors and their relative consistency in each of the comparisons (group, time, groups by time) provides a measure of confidence in the reliability and validity of TAI scores for assessing intervention effects.

DISCUSSION

Emergency Room Simulator[33] is a single-user computer-based simulation designed to provide experiential learning in a safe environment. The program reinforces prior learning on prioritizing acuity levels of patients presenting to the emergency room and improved clinical judgments as measured by cognitive gain (accuracy) and time to decision (efficiency). The design of the program supports ELT through concrete clinical experience, time for reflection, and comprehension followed by feedback on active experimentation (decision making).

There were limitations to the study. The sample size was small, and to generalize these findings and determine the program's efficacy the intervention should be tested with larger samples of senior nursing students. Because of the small sample, there was insufficient variability for testing differences in education, race, or gender. Students saw a similar test (the pretest) and although the clinical scenarios varied, some may have scored better the second time regardless of the intervention. Experiential learning occurs over time and should be tested over a longer period to determine the retention of knowledge, which would further support Kolb's theory that learning is experiential and transformative. Efficiency may be related to confidence, and additional research that seeks confidence levels of the participants would be beneficial in determining the efficacy of the intervention. The instrument was new, and additional testing to determine validity and reliability is needed.

IMPLICATIONS FOR ELT IN NURSE EDUCATION

Nurses are often the first point of contact with patients in high-acuity areas. Their clinical judgment must be accurate and efficient; however, clinical judgment requires reflection on concrete experiences to shape understanding and build critical thinking skills. Nurse educators may find it difficult to provide the needed breadth and depth of experience for their students in the actual clinical setting. Although other forms of simulation, such as high-fidelity patient simulators, offer educational opportunities, they are expensive and time intensive. The use of computer-based simulation, such as Emergency Room Simulator, as an adjunctive learning strategy provides experiential learning that is available as often and at any time desired. Computer-based simulation or similar programs may serve as a valuable resource for nurse educators seeking alternative ways to increase clinical judgment skills in the prelicensure nursing student. It may also be used in the workplace to enhance the clinical judgment of existing registered nurses. Additional testing may include using the simulation for registered nurses interested in emergency triage.

SUMMARY

Experiential learning, such as computer-based simulation, promises to be a valuable tool for increasing clinical judgment skills. The use of case studies has long been used in education, and incorporating this teaching/learning strategy into an interactive, autonomous computer-based simulation offers an additional aid in potentially enhancing clinical judgment. Availability of Internet-based programs through work, college, or personal computers makes the simulation experience easily accessible to learners. According to this initial pilot study, the software program Emergency Room Simulator holds promise as an innovative computer-based experiential learning strategy to promote clinical judgment skills in a safe and easily accessible format. Additional testing is needed on this and other computer screen–based experiential learning programs. This study contributes to knowledge in health care research by suggesting innovations that have promise in developing clinical judgment skills through experiential learning.

ACKNOWLEDGMENTS

The author would like to acknowledge and thank Dr Michael Allen, Vice Provost for Research and Dean of the College of Graduate Studies, Middle Tennessee State University, for funding this pilot study.

REFERENCES

1. Banning M. Nursing research: perspectives on critical thinking. Br J Nurs 2006; 15(8):458–61.
2. Facione PA, Facione DH. Externalizing the critical thinking in knowledge development and clinical judgment. Nurs Outlook 1996;44:129–36.
3. Kuiper RA, Pesut DJ. Promoting cognitive and metacognitive reflective reasoning skills in nursing practice: self-regulated learning theory. J Adv Nurs 2004;45: 381–91.
4. Jenkins SD. Cross-cultural perspectives on critical thinking. J Nurs Educ 2011; 50(5). http://dx.doi.org/10.3928/01484834–20110228–02.
5. Roche JP. A pilot study of teaching clinical decision making with the clinical educator model. J Nurs Educ 2002;41:365–7.
6. Lauri S, Salantera S. Developing an instrument to measure and describe clinical decision making in different nursing fields. J Prof Nurs 2002;18:93–100.
7. Del Bueno D. A crisis in critical thinking. Nurs Educ Perspect 2005;26(5):278–82.
8. Jeffries PR. A framework for designing, implementing, and evaluating simulations used as teaching strategies in nursing. Nurs Educ Perspect 2005;26(2):96–102.
9. Daly WM. The development of an alternative method in the assessment of critical thinking as an outcome of nursing education. J Adv Nurs 2001;36(1):120–30.

10. Myrick F, Yonge F. Enhancing critical thinking in the preceptorship experience in nursing education. J Adv Nurs 2004;45(4):371–80.
11. Benner P, Tanner C, Chesla C. Expertise in nursing practice: caring, clinical judgment, and ethics. 2nd edition. New York: Springer; 2009.
12. Benner P. From novice to expert. Am J Nurs 1982;82:402–7.
13. Overstreet ML. The current practice of nursing clinical simulation debriefing: a multiple case study (Doctoral dissertation). 2009. Available at: http://trace. tennessee.edu/cgi/viewcontent.cgi?article=1696&context=utk_graddiss. Accessed August 8, 2012.
14. Kolb DA. Experiential learning: experience as the source of learning and development. Englewood Cliffs (NJ): Prentice-Hall; 1984.
15. Gaba D. A brief history of mannequin-based simulation & application (2004). In: Dunn W, editor. Simulators in critical care and beyond. Des Plaines (IL): Society of Critical Care Medicine; 2001. p. 7–14.
16. Jeffries P, Rogers K. Theoretical frameworks for simulation design. Chapter 3. In: Jeffries P, editor. Simulation in nursing education. New York: National League of Nursing; 2007. p. 21–33.
17. Medley C, Horne C. Using simulation technology for undergraduate nursing education. J Nurs Educ 2005;44(1):31–4.
18. Dobbs C, Sweitzer V, Jeffries P. Testing simulation design features using an insulin management simulation in nursing education. Clinical Simulation in Nursing 2006;2(1):e17–22.
19. Toomy MA. Learning with cases. J Contin Educ Nurs 2003;34(1):34–8.
20. DeYoung S. Teaching strategies for nurse educators. Upper Saddle River (NJ): Prentis Hall; 2003.
21. Bentley GW. Problem-based learning. In: Lowenstein AJ, Bradshaw MJ, editors. Fuszard's innovative teaching strategies in nursing. 3rd edition. Gaithersburg (MD): Aspen; 2001. p. 83–106.
22. White MJ, Amos E, Kouzekanani K. Problem-based learning: an outcomes student. Nurse Educ 1999;24(2):33–6.
23. Werth EP, Werth L. Effective training for millennial students. Adult Learn 2011; 22(3):12–9.
24. Suave L, Renaud L, Kaufman D, et al. Distinguishing between games and simulations: a systematic review. Educ Tech Soc 2007;10(3). http://dx.doi.org/ 10.1.1.169.5559.
25. Dieterle E. Multi-user virtual environments for teaching and learning. In: Pagani M, editor. Encyclopedia of multimedia technology and networking. 2nd edition. Hershey (PA): Idea Group, Inc; 2009. p. 1033–41.
26. Kilmon CA, Brown L, Ghosh S, et al. Immersive virtual reality simulations in nursing education. Nurs Educ Perspect 2010;31(5):314–7.
27. Royse MA, Newton SE. How gaming is used as an innovative strategy for nursing education. Nurs Educ Perspect 2007;28(5):263–7.
28. Porter JE. Nurse triage. BMJ 1993;306:208–9.
29. Robertson-Steel I. Evolution of triage systems. Emerg Med J 2006;23(2):154–5.
30. Qureshi NA. Triage systems: a review of the literature with reference to Saudi Arabia. Eastern Mediterranean Health Journal 2010;16(6):690–8.
31. Considine J, Lucas E, Martin R, et al. Rapid intervention and treatment zone: redesigning nursing services to meet increasing emergency department demand. Int J Nurs Pract 2012;18:60–7.
32. Moreschi D, Moreschi C. (Producer). Triage in the emergency department [Software]. 2010. Available at: http://swiftriveronline.com. Accessed August 8, 2012.

33. Gilboy N, Tanabe P, Travers DA, et al. Emergency severity index, version 4: implementation handbook. AHRQ Publication No. 05-0046-2. Rockville (MD): Agency for Healthcare Research and Quality; 2005.
34. Nitko AJ. Educational assessment of students. 3rd edition. Upper Saddle River (NJ): Prentice-Hall; 2001.
35. Herrman JW. Keeping their attention: innovative strategies for nursing education. J Contin Educ Nurs 2011;42(10):449–56. http://dx.doi.org/10.3928/00220124–20110516–05.

Transdisciplinary Simulation
Learning and Practicing Together

Kymberlee Montgomery, DrNP, APRN, WHNP-BC, CNE[a],*,
Sharon Griswold-Theodorson, MD, MPH[b],
Kate Morse, APRN, ACNP-BC[c], Owen Montgomery, MD[d],
Dana Farabaugh, MD[d]

KEYWORDS

- Transdisciplinary simulation • Interprofessional education • Collaboration

KEY POINTS

- The Institute of Medicine, partnering with national private foundations, has challenged existing approaches to health care delivery and patient safety by suggesting a redesign of the U.S. health care system.
- This article explores the historical and philosophic imperative to change health care education to a seamless transdisciplinary model to foster interprofessional communication and collaboration during the formative training years.
- To improve patient safety and quality of care and reduce medical error, students in health care disciplines will need to be educated together to practice together effectively.

INTRODUCTION

The provision of quality safe care in the complex health care arena of the twenty-first century requires the use of an integrated team approach on a daily basis across all care spectrums. Teams and clinicians in health care systems face obstacles daily that impact the overall quality of the care provided. These obstacles include fiscal challenges, increased liability in response to patient safety errors, and work force issues. Clinicians and clinical care teams are managing a rapidly aging population

Disclosures: None of the authors has a relationship with a commercial company that has a direct financial interest in the subject matter or materials discussed in the article.
[a] Nurse Practitioner Programs, Drexel University College of Nursing and Health Professions, Drexel University College of Medicine, MS 501 Bellet Building 725, 1505 Race Street, Philadelphia, PA 19102, USA; [b] Department of Emergency Medicine, Drexel University College of Medicine, Room 2108, 2nd Floor, MS 1011 NCB, 245 North 15th Street, Philadelphia, PA 19102, USA; [c] Department of Nursing, Drexel University College of Nursing and Health Professions, MS 501 Bellet Building 827, 1505 Race Street, Philadelphia, PA 19102, USA; [d] Department of Obstetrics and Gynecology, Drexel University College of Medicine, 245 North 15th Street, MS 495 NCB, Philadelphia, PA 19102, USA
* Corresponding author.
E-mail address: Kae33@drexel.edu

with its increasingly complex and compounded chronic health problems while, at the same time, are expected to incorporate ever-evolving health care technologies. For a large part of the U.S. population, health care inequities and limited access to care further compound an overburdened health care response system. The Patient Protection and Affordable Care Act (PPACA)[1] and the Health Care and Education Reconciliation Act,[2] both heralded as the most significant health care reforms of the past 3 decades, were designed to address and ameliorate many of these obstacles. The PPACA legislation mandates the use of coordinated interdisciplinary clinical teams to deliver higher quality care in a more cost-effective manner to a larger number of previously uninsured Americans (estimated >30 million) who will gain insurance with this legislation. The PPACA and the Health Care and Education Reconciliation Act of 2010 provide the opportunity and responsibility for health care academic institutions to redesign existing health care curricula and create new paradigms for training in interprofessional team-based care.[1,2]

Although patient care must always occur with health care teams working together, it is a paradox in current educational models that each discipline educates and trains its providers in its own individual "silo." Schools of nursing, health care professions, and medicine can exist on the same campus, but they rarely collaborate and integrate the learning experiences of their students. Oftentimes, students do not understand the importance of communication and team collaboration until they enter practice as a novice clinician. They often feel unprepared in the skill sets necessary to work together in the continually changing and challenging clinical setting. To promote collaboration, improve patient quality of care and safety, and increase communication within the health care delivery systems, education of health care professionals needs to change: to practice better together, we need to learn together.

BACKGROUND AND SIGNIFICANCE

A national recommendation for interprofessional education is not new and did not evolve from health care reform. The roots for this call for a transformation can be traced back 4 decades. In 1972, the Institute of Medicine (IOM) convened the first national forum on interprofessional education in health care in the United States.[3] The conclusions of the conference were aimed at 3 aspects of the challenge to health care educators: administrative, teaching, and national. The committee stressed the importance of recognizing the obligation to engage in interdisciplinary education, the value of clinical settings for developing interdisciplinary education, and the need for governmental and professional support of interdisciplinary education for health care delivery teams.[3] Although this report continues to be as compelling today as it was 40 years ago, the conclusions have not become the reality of today's health care educational institutions.

The landmark 1999 IOM report "To Err is Human: Building a Safer Health System"[4] and its companion report "Crossing the Quality Chasm: A New Health System for the 21st Century"[5] reported as many as 98,000 deaths per year from medical errors, uncovering significant quality and safety issues plaguing the health care system. Increased technological opportunities, coupled with this newly uncovered awareness, pressured government and academia to begin the challenge to the current "siloed" educational processes by "placing more stress on teaching evidence-based practice and providing more opportunities for interdisciplinary training."[5(pp6)] Three years later, an IOM multidisciplinary committee continued to ignite educational changes through "Health Professions Education: A Bridge to Quality."[6] This report reiterated the need for all health care professionals to be educated to deliver patient-centered care as members of an interdisciplinary team, emphasizing evidence-based practice, quality improvement approaches, and informatics. It took 7 more years of mounting pressure to build a unified consensus among governmental and private foundations to transform the health care and health education systems in the United States. This pressure included the escalating governmental spending (cost) for less-than-optimal quality; a growing number of uninsured Americans with poor access to care; and the increasing fear of the middle class population's inability to afford basic health care services.

The second decade of the twenty-first century began with the greatest promise of change: the passage of health care reform and the publication of 3 sentinel reports from the most respected organizations in the world. In the IOM's report "The Future of Nursing: Leading Change, Advancing Health,"[7] for the first time, the nursing profession is elevated to equal status as a partner in the development of health care in the United States. In addition, to be an integral part of the solution to the health care crisis, nurses must be encouraged to practice to the full extent of their training. The World Health Organization's (WHO) "Framework for Action on Interprofessional Education and Collaborative Practice" echoes the IOM report regarding nurses' central position in health care, and concludes that after almost 50 years of enquiry, "Evidence is insufficient to indicate that effective interprofessional education enables effective collaborative practice."[8(pp7)] Lastly, a global independent commission on the Education of Health Professionals for the 21st Century coordinated by the Harvard School of Public Health published "Transforming Education to Strengthen Health Systems in an Interdependent World."[9] This substantial report proposes that educational reform should promote interprofessional and transprofessional education and nonhierarchical relationships in effective teams. One hundred years after the publication of the Flexner[10] report in 1910, the time has come for a new generation of health care education reform for the global health care problems.

In 2011, 40 years after the initial IOM call to action for collaboration among health care professionals, 6 of the major national health care organizations finally convened an expert panel to produce documents containing the foundation of interprofessional education. "Team-Based Competencies: Building a Shared Foundation for Education and Clinical Practice"[11] and "Core Competencies for Interprofessional Collaborative Practice: Report of an Expert Panel"[12] define 4 measurable core competency domains and 38 subcompetencies for curriculum foundation for interprofessional education and practice in all health care realms:

- Values/ethics for interprofessional practice
- Roles/responsibilities
- Interprofessional communication
- Teams and teamwork

Medicine, nursing, public health, pharmacy, and dentistry in collaboration with Health Resource Service Administration (HRSA)[11,12] and representatives of major foundations created the groundwork for the action plan to use these competencies to transform health care education and health care delivery. "The status quo of educating health professionals in silos without preparing them for the current realities of everyday practice is no longer tenable."[11(pp9)]

LESSONS LEARNED

During a transdisciplinary clinical simulation of a high-risk obstetric scenario at a major university academic center, Resident X, an occasionally overconfident

*third year obstetrics/gynecology resident, has just successfully completed a simu-
lated vaginal delivery of a full-term infant complicated by shoulder dystocia. Resident X breathes an overly proud sigh of relief as the successfully delivered infant is
quickly passed off to the neonatal team. Understandably, the attention of the
simulated clinical team turns to the compromised infant. The crew chief directing
the case from the control room instructs the standardized patient through an
earpiece to start the simulated hemorrhage. As the profuse bleeding begins
and the patient's blood pressure drops, Resident X, left alone at the bedside, realizes that he and his patient are in jeopardy. Fully engaged in the simulation, he
spontaneously and in earnest screams, "I NEED A NURSE!"*

Health care professionals recognize that clinical care, in both ambulatory and acute
settings, is most effectively delivered in teams. From this digitally recorded and
debriefed real educational exercise, all participants identified crucial messages
regarding team communication, quality of patient care, and patient safety. Resident
X learned that the physician alone is not sufficient for the provision of health care,
particularly in complicated scenarios. The team representatives from undergraduate
nursing students, physician assistant students, nurse anesthesia students, anesthesia
residents, confederate nurses, midwives, and physicians realized that without each
team member possessing an understanding of one's own roles and responsibilities,
and those of the collective team, the patient, the team members, and the team itself
are compromised and left vulnerable to error. The interprofessional educators who
designed, observed, and debriefed the simulated experience further recognized the
importance of interprofessional team-based scenarios and enhanced their commitment to embed interprofessional education early in the curriculum design across all
health care disciplines (**Box 1**).

EVIDENCE TO SUPPORT HOW INTERPROFESSIONAL EDUCATION IMPROVES PATIENT OUTCOMES

The WHO[8] has suggested a roadmap to illustrate how interprofessional educational
efforts support positive outcomes in real-life scenarios and programs around the
country, and are turning ideas into stories of success. Much of the research shows
that adverse events in patient management in the hospital setting are often associated
with 2 recurrent problems: (1) poor communication[13] or teamwork climate,[14,15] and (2)
gaps in a provider's technical skills or knowledge base. Improved teamwork climate
and effective communication among health care providers can be defined as nontechnical skills (NTS). Several articles have begun to show how transdisciplinary team
training can positively impact clinical outcomes via improvement in NTS. Some of
the greatest clinical impact articles from a variety of clinical specialties are highlighted
here.

Siassakos and colleagues[16] studied teamwork in the United Kingdom extensively.
This research group was among the first to stress that improved clinical outcomes
can be demonstrated after implementation of simulation-based, obstetric-specific
training interventions in conjunction with teamwork training. Specifically after conducting a series of multicenter, prospective controlled trials, they found that improved
teamwork behavior was more likely to be associated with timely administration of
appropriate dosages of magnesium, an essential medication in the treatment of
eclampsia.[16,17]

Draycott and colleagues[18] were among the first to show that multidisciplinary simulation training resulted in an improved clinical outcome in the hospital setting. The
introduction of mandatory obstetric emergencies training courses for nurse midwives

Box 1
Transdisciplinary delivery room scenario guide

Learning objectives

Demonstrate effective communication in an emergency setting within team

Demonstrate effective communication with consults called

Demonstrate the available and appropriate resources to call in an emergency

Communicate in a therapeutic manner with the patient and family

Recognize cardiopulmonary event leading to Disseminated Intervascular Coagulation (DIC) Amniotic Fluid Embolism (AFE)

Demonstrate management of Airway, Breathing, Circulation (ABCs)

Identify appropriate fluid and product replacement

Materials needed

Live patient with prompt birther attached

Blood for hemorrhage: red and blue if available

Fetal monitor

Maternal cardiac monitor

Code cart available

Hemorrhage medications: cytotec, pitocin, methergine, hemabate

Obstetrical Scenario

Prebrief: change of shift

27-year-old G5P3013 at 39 + 2 weeks just arrived in active labor; uncomplicated prenatal care; fetal heart rate in 150s; checked in triage: 8 cm/+2 and membranes still intact; moved to labor room.

Called to room for delivery

Patient claims " the baby is coming, it's coming. I think my water just broke"

Vitals: blood pressure 130/85, pulse 110, pulse oximetry reveals 99% on room air

Fetal monitor: rate in the 150s; early decelerations noted; contractions every 1 to 2 minutes

Patient undergoes normal vaginal delivery; infant handed off to pediatrics team

During delivery patient begins complaining of chest pain

Oxygen saturation levels drop to 82% on room air, pulse 60, blood pressure 80/40

Patient minimally responsive and bleeding vaginally

Team Objectives

Team should recognize cardiopulmonary event and begin resuscitative measures

Intravenous access, intravenous fluids

Call anesthesia (potentially rapid response team; not code team)

Mental status deteriorates to unresponsive

Team member communicates with family

Team should recognize hemorrhage/potential DIC

Call for hemorrhage kit demonstrates knowledge of correct medications, usage, dose, and route of administration

Laboratory tests: complete blood cell count, coagulations, type and cross, tryptase (if the team is really on top of it, that is the test they would ask for)

Team should recognize 2 indications for intubation:

1. Loss of ability to protect patient's airway when mental status deteriorates

2. Inability to oxygenate with supplemental noninvasive support

Patient will need an ABG or arterial line because pulse oximetry will not work while her blood pressure continues to drop

Blood replacement: recognize that factors will also need to be replaced, not just red blood cells

Recommend notifying intensive care unit

Request bedside echocardiogram

Scenario will end once patient is stabilized: ABCs have been addressed; intensive care unit notified; fluid and product replacement has been initiated

and physician staff were associated with a significant reduction in low 5-min Apgar scores and hypoxic ischemic encephalopathy (HIE) in newborns. The training was continued and the improvement in Apgar scores and decreased incidence of HIE was sustained. This important study documented one of the first occasions that an educational simulation intervention was shown to be associated with a clinically important, and sustained, improvement in perinatal outcomes.

Since the landmark Draycott and colleagues[18] article, Riley and colleagues[19] showed that a simulation-based intervention in addition to interdisciplinary team training resulted in a statistically significant 37% improvement in a perinatal morbidity score. The authors used the Weighted Adverse Outcome Score (WAOS) measure of perinatal morbidity and a culture of safety survey (safety attitudes questionnaire) pre-intervention and postintervention to compare 3 hospital groups. The first group served as a control, the second group received the U.S. Agency for Healthcare Research and Quality's (AHRQ) supported curriculum (TeamSTEPPS training,[20] a didactic training program), and the third group received the TeamSTEPPS program combined with a series of in situ simulation training exercises. The authors concluded that a comprehensive interdisciplinary team training program using in situ simulation in addition to transdisciplinary team training in NTS can improve perinatal safety in the hospital setting. They also reinforced that didactic instruction alone without simulation was not effective in improving perinatal outcomes.

Similar findings have also been shown in disciplines other than maternal fetal health. In 2010 Capella and colleagues[21] studied trauma team performance and its affect on clinical outcomes after simulation-based training and instruction in essential team competencies based on TeamSTEPPS training.[20] Clinical outcomes and team performance assessments were evaluated during trauma resuscitations observed preintervention and postintervention. Nurses, residents, and faculty attended a 2-hour didactic session to review roles and responsibilities followed by additional multidisciplinary simulation sessions that reinforced knowledge transfer and teamwork communication. The authors reported that time to CT, time to endotracheal intubation, and time to operating room were all significantly improved after training. This important study has demonstrated that teamwork training led to improved teamwork performance, which resulted in improved clinical care during trauma resuscitations.

Armed with affirmation in the literature, redefined well articulated core competencies, and the imperative to transform the education of health professions, Drexel University's interprofessional education (IPE) team was charged with developing curriculum that encompasses the 4 domains and the subcompetencies. Several universities have begun interprofessional education initiatives unique to the needs of their programs and their faculty.

THE DREXEL IPEC

Drexel is a nationally certified Center of Excellence for Women's Health. In 2008, Drexel University's College of Nursing and Health Professions and College of Medicine partnered together to create innovative transdisciplinary health care education initiatives commencing early on in the respective women's health curricula. Although many initiatives use terms such as *interdisciplinary*, *multidisciplinary*, and *transdisciplinary* to describe collaborative programmatic efforts, the term *transdisciplinary* was purposefully selected at Drexel to convey the commitment of the participants to strive to develop sufficient trust and mutual confidence to transcend disciplinary boundaries and adopt a more comprehensive approach.[22] Women's health programs at Drexel are a natural vehicle for transdisciplinary education. Sharing a wealth of knowledge and clinical expertise, nurse practitioners, certified nurse midwives, students, physicians, and physician assistants use didactic seminars and low-fidelity simulation to instruct medical students about the importance of disease prevention and health promotion regarding the health care of women. For most medical students, this is the initial point of exposure to instruction by disciplines other than basic scientists and medicine.

The major focus of interprofessional education at Drexel is the Transdisciplinary Simulation Initiative. Using the aforementioned core competencies, this innovative educational program has combined diverse expert faculty instruction, multilevel simulation, and collaborative case study formatting to residents and nurse practitioner, nurse anesthesia, physician assistant, and undergraduate nursing students together in a transdisciplinary women's health setting. Shoulder dystocia, postpartum hemorrhage, eclampsia, amniotic fluid embolism, airway compromise, uterine and ovarian disorders, pelvic pain, ectopic pregnancy, pelvic inflammatory disease, vaginal infections, and birth control–related thromboembolism are medical complications that frequently challenge health care teams working in obstetrics and gynecology departments and emergency rooms.[23] These challenges are threaded through the case studies and simulated scenarios in Drexel's program. In addition, the transdisciplinary teams simulate difficult conversations with standardized patients (SP), which include giving bad news, taking a thorough sexual history, and participating in ethical decision-making scenarios; the teams then receive real-time feedback from the SP and clinical faculty. Initially funded by the Robert Wood Johnson Executive Nurse Fellows program, the purpose of this endeavor has been to enhance knowledge of roles and responsibilities in the health care system, foster the development of team building skills, improve health care team communication, reduce medical error, and increase patient safety and quality of care. Preliminary data suggest significant increases in collaborative attitudes for mutual support and communication within the transdisciplinary teams.[24]

At the conclusion of each scenario, key faculty members debrief the transdisciplinary team. These faculty members are from each of the disciplines and have been trained in the "Debriefing with Good Judgment" model[25] by The Center for Medical Simulation at Harvard University. Group debriefing after participation in simulation exercises contributes to the richness of the simulated experience; furthermore, it is critical to acknowledge the students' perspective, explore participant decisions and actions in greater detail, and link the experience to authentic patient care. The literature suggests that well-structured debriefing yields the greatest educational experiences.[25–29]

Engaging students in reflective exercises is a complex but worthwhile endeavor. Therefore, debriefing, which requires active engagement on the part of faculty and learners, is clearly differentiated from feedback, which can be more passive.

Planning for debriefing begins with the initial planning of the simulation scenario and should be guided by the learning objectives for the exercise. Preparation for debriefing interprofessional health care simulations requires an interprofessional debriefing team to ensure that all students are actively engaged in the process. The risks of having a single-specialty debriefer address an transdisciplinary team include a narrow scope of discussion, lack of understanding all team members' perspectives, and discomfort in exploring the actions and thought processes of people in other specialties, all of which can result in disengagement of some learners.

SUMMARY AND FUTURE VISIONS

Clearly, exciting and unique programs like Drexel's exist in multiple institutions in the United States and around the world. These academic health centers have chosen many different educational vehicles to attempt to achieve the same shared vision. This shared vision of global health care includes a workforce in which

1. Present and future health care providers will be educated using a competency-based transdisciplinary health care curriculum;
2. Health care providers are educated in teams and are "collaborative practice–ready" when they enter clinical practice; and
3. Team-driven collaborative practices improve the health care services provided to patients, strengthen the health systems, and continue to improve health outcomes.

The authors have substantial experience with highly successful team-based collaborative practices and innovative transdisciplinary educational experiences, and they share this vision for an improved future health care system.

In addition, the authors challenge the current innovators, foundations, health profession organizations, and governmental agencies to contribute additional rigor and research to the educational program developmental process. To help new programs learn how to overcome the multiple barriers to working and learning together, it is absolutely necessary to have a "national clearinghouse" for innovative transdisciplinary educational programs, as IOM requested in the 1972 report[1] (and again in the 2010 IPEC report[8]). However, a clearinghouse of successful individual transdisciplinary programs, though necessary, is not sufficient to direct the correct and sustainable changes that must occur in both the educational and clinical domains. Sound curricula must be the driving force for any innovative transdisciplinary program. As with any scientific endeavor proposing major change, the evidence-based outcome measurements of initial transdisciplinary interventions and the rigorous "debriefing" of educational programs must be available before the innovative programs can be accepted as the new standards.

The changes the authors have successfully implemented within their institution have been the result of sustained persistent efforts championed by leadership throughout the institution. Successful implementation of an interprofessional curriculum is charged with challenges that must be overcome, the foremost of which is the ability to change the culture in which health care providers are educated. The work of the transdisciplinary innovators, academic health care profession community, and IPEC is incomplete until the outcomes of competencies can be measured and the new curriculum can be built based on the knowledge that public health has been truly improved.

ACKNOWLEDGMENTS

The authors would like to acknowledge the leadership and support of Dr MaryEllen Glasgow, PhD, RN, ACNS-BC, Robert Wood Johnson (RWJ) Foundation Executive Nurse Fellow. Her RWJ project, *Educating Professional Nurses for Tomorrow's Complex Clinical Environment & Emerging Demographics: Enhancing Safety & Inter-Professional Communication* further transdisciplinary simulation endeavors at Drexel University into reality.

REFERENCES

1. Patient Care and Affordable Care Act (2010) (PPACA) USC § 42 USC 18001 (2010).
2. Health Care and Reconciliation Act (2010) USC § 42 2372a (2010).
3. Institute of Medicine. Educating for the health team. Available at: http://www. ipe.umn.edu/prod/groups/ahc/@pub/@ahc/@cipe/documents/asset/ahc_asset_ 350123.pdf. Accessed May 4, 2012.
4. Institute of Medicine. To err is human: building a safer health system. Available at: http://www.nap.edu/openbook.php?isbn=0309068371. Accessed May 4, 2012.
5. Institute of Medicine. Crossing the quality chasm: a new health system for the 21st century. Available at: http://iom.edu/Reports/2001/Crossing-the-Quality-Chasm-A-New-Health-System-for-the-21st-Century.aspx. Accessed April 29, 2012.
6. Institute of Medicine. Health professions education: a bridge to quality. Available at: http://www.iom.edu/Reports/2003/Health-Professions-Education-A-Bridge-to-Quality.aspx. Accessed May 2, 2012.
7. Institute of Medicine. The future of nursing: leading change, advancing health. Available at: http://www.iom.edu/Reports/2010/The-Future-of-Nursing-Leading-Change-Advancing-Health.aspx. Accessed May 4, 2012.
8. Collaborative practice. Available at: http://www.who.int/hrh/nursing_midwifery/en/. Accessed May 6, 2012.
9. Frenk J, Chen L, Bhutta Z, et al. Health professionals for a new century: transforming education to strengthen health systems in an interdependent world. Lancet 2010;376:1923–58.
10. Flexner A. Medical education in the United States and Canada: a report to the Carnegie Foundation for the advancement of teaching. New York: Carnegie Foundation for the Advancement of Teaching; 1910.
11. Team-based competencies: building a shared foundation for education and clinical practice. Available at: http://library.med.utah.edu/ipe/resources/team-based_ competencies.pdf. Accessed August 1, 2012.
12. Interprofessional Education Collaborative Expert Panel. Core competencies for interprofessional collaborative practice: report of an expert panel. Washington, DC: Interprofessional Education Collaborative; 2011.
13. Salas E, Wilson KA, Murphy CE, et al. Communicating, coordinating, and cooperating when lives depend on it: tips for teamwork. Jt Comm J Qual Patient Saf 2008;34(6):333–41.
14. Pronovost PJ, Berenholtz SM, Goeschel C, et al. Improving patient safety in intensive care units in Michigan. J Crit Care 2008;23(2):207–21.
15. Rabol LI, Ostergaard D, Mogensen T. Outcomes of classroom-based team training interventions for multiprofessional hospital staff. A systematic review. Qual Saf Health Care 2010;19(6):469–596.
16. Siassakos D, Bristowe K, Draycott TJ, et al. Clinical efficiency in a simulated emergency and relationship to team behaviours: a multisite cross-sectional study. BJOG 2011;118(5):596–607.

17. Siassakos D, Fox R, Crofts JF, et al. The management of a simulated emergency: better teamwork, better performance. Resuscitation 2011;82(2):203–6.
18. Draycott T, Sibanda T, Owen L, et al. Does training in obstetric emergencies improve neonatal outcome? BJOG 2006;113(2):177–82.
19. Riley W, Davis S, Miller K, et al. Didactic and simulation nontechnical skills team training to improve perinatal patient outcomes in a community hospital. Jt Comm J Qual Patient Saf 2011;37(8):357–64.
20. TeamSTEPPS. Agency for Healthcare Research and Quality Web site. Available at: http://teamstepps.ahrq.gov. Accessed May 7, 2012.
21. Capella J, Smith S, Philp A, et al. Teamwork training improves the clinical care of trauma patients. J Surg Educ 2010;67(6):439–43.
22. Choi B, Pak A. Multidisciplinarity, interdisciplinarity and transdisciplinarity in health research, services, education, and policy: definitions, objectives, and evidence of effectiveness. Clin Invest Med 2006;29(6):351–64.
23. Montgomery K, Morse K, Smith-Glasgow ME, et al. Promoting quality and safety in women's health through the use of transdisciplinary clinical simulation modules: methodology and a pilot trial. Gend Med 2012;9(15):S48–54.
24. Posmontier B, Montgomery K, Smith-Glasgow ME, et al. Transdisciplinary teamwork simulation in obstetrics-gynecology health care. J Nurs Educ 2012;51(3): 176–9.
25. Rudolph J, Simon R, Rivard P, et al. Debriefing with good judgement: combining rigorous feedback with genuine inquiry. Anesthesiol Clin 2007;25(2):361–76.
26. Cantrell MA. Clinical Simulation in Nursing Education. Clin Sim Nurs 2008;4: e19–23.
27. Brackenreg J. Issues in reflection and debriefing: how nurse educators structure experiential activities. Nurse Educ Pract 2004;4(4):264–70.
28. Fanning RM, Gaba DM. The role of debriefing in simulation-based learning. Simul Healthc 2007;2(2):115–25.
29. Gordon CJ, Buckley T. The effect of high-fidelity simulation training on medical-surgical graduate nurses' perceived ability to respond to patient clinical emergencies. J Contin Educ Nurs 2009;40(11):491–500.

Learning from Business
Incorporating the Toyota Production System into Nursing Curricula

Joanne Farley Serembus, EdD, RN, CCRN, CNE[a],*,
Faye Meloy, PhD, MSN, MBA, RN[b],
Bobbie Posmontier, PhD, CNM, PMHNP-BC[c]

KEYWORDS

• Toyota Production System • Lean organization • Nursing curricula

KEY POINTS

- Drexel University investigated a new nursing education model designed to prepare nurses to excel in a complex health care environment, as well as to foster leadership skills, interprofessional collaboration, evidence-based lifelong learning, and critical thinking skills.
- Faculty looked to the Toyota Production System (TPS), as it had established credibility in both industry and health care settings.
- Drexel University is the first academic institution to incorporate the principles of the TPS into nursing education.

In 2010, the United States government ushered in the most radical transformation in health care delivery since 1965 with the passage of the Patient Affordable Care Act, which addressed improving patient outcomes and access to care for all Americans.[1] In response to the challenge, members of the Robert Wood Johnson Foundation (RWJF) partnered with members of the Institute of Medicine (IOM) and charted the future of nursing in their collaborative report *The Future of Nursing: Leading Change, Advancing Health.*[2] This visionary group understood that nurses, who comprise the largest group of health professionals caring for patients, have the greatest impact

Funding: This article was completed as part of a grant from the Robert Wood Johnson Foundation.
[a] College of Nursing and Health Professions, Drexel University, 1505 Race Street, Mail Stop 501, Bellet Building Room 1027, Philadelphia, PA 19102, USA; [b] Pre-licensure BSN Programs, BSN Co-op Department, College of Nursing and Health Professions, Drexel University, 1505 Race Street, MS 501, Bellet Building Room 727, Philadelphia, PA 19102, USA; [c] College of Nursing and Health Professions, Drexel University, 1505 Race Street, MS 1030, Bellet Building Room 524, Philadelphia, PA 19102, USA
* Corresponding author.
E-mail address: jmf64@drexel.edu

Nurs Clin N Am 47 (2012) 503–516
http://dx.doi.org/10.1016/j.cnur.2012.07.005
0029-6465/12/$ – see front matter © 2012 Elsevier Inc. All rights reserved.

on patient outcomes and are the vital link between access to care and quality outcomes. In addition, the members understood that nurses play a pivotal role in preventing medical errors, increasing patient safety, reducing infection, decreasing fragmentation of services, and providing holistic, culturally sensitive, ethical, and compassionate care.

One of the most salient recommendations was to transform nursing education curricula to better facilitate the emergence of a sufficient pool of highly qualified nursing graduates, who would be capable of caring for patients across the life span with increasingly complex health care needs within a highly technological environment.[2] It was further recommended that nursing curricula should promote a student-centered, competency-based learning environment as delineated by the American Association of Colleges of Nursing (AACN) that facilitates the emergence of nursing graduates with exemplary leadership skills, interprofessional collaboration, entrepreneurial and business savvy, evidence-based lifelong learning, and critical thinking skills.[3] This new skill set would serve to improve the transition of nursing graduates from academic settings to practice, to better serve the needs of patients and reduce medical error.

After learning of Virginia Mason Medical Center's successful adaptation of the Toyota Production System (TPS) in the health care setting, faculty at Drexel University College of Nursing and Health Professions (CNHP) embarked on a journey of incorporating TPS principles into its nursing curriculum. The goal was to lay a foundation in support of curricular reform to prepare nursing graduates capable of working effectively in a complex health care environment. The purpose of this article is to share the journey of transformation, the application of TPS principles as a means of bridging the gap between education and practice, and the lessons learned in the process.

BACKGROUND

The landmark reports from the IOM *To Err is Human* and *Crossing the Quality Chasm* sounded the alarm that thousands of people die unnecessarily or are harmed each year because of medical mistakes and ineffective health care delivery models.[4,5] In addition to the human cost of these problems, the IOM also estimated that medical mistakes result in an estimated $17 billion to $29 billion per year of additional costs to a health care system already overburdened with significant resource constraints. The IOM reports suggest that in the United States "health care harms too frequently and routinely fails to deliver its potential benefits."[5] As a result, governmental agencies, payers, health care accrediting bodies, professional associations, and the public are unified in the call for health care reform with an emphasis on decreasing adverse patient outcomes and development of high-quality, cost-effective health care delivery models. Although specific strategies were developed by the Institute for Healthcare Improvement (IHI), the Agency for Health Research and Quality (AHRQ), The Joint Commission, and professional organizations to reduce medical error and improve patient outcomes, progress in eliminating preventable medical errors has been slow and inconsistent. The IOM report *To Err is Human* also suggested that medical mistakes are not the fault of "bad people" but rather the result of ineffective "systems" that fail to identify potential defects before problems occur.[5] Increasingly the lack of progress has been attributed to an overreliance on "fixes" and isolated outcome benchmarks rather than on purposeful development of a shared vision and culture of safety complemented by fail-safe systems in every aspect of the patient health care encounter.[6] Health care providers are gradually putting aside professional silos and elitism to look outside the traditional boundaries of health care solutions to find innovations that will enhance quality, safety, and cost-effectiveness of patient care. The TPS, which has enjoyed success in the automotive, aviation, and nuclear industries, is one of these unique innovations that have produced profoundly positive results in the health care industry.[7]

THE TOYOTA PRODUCTION SYSTEM

The TPS principles, derived from one of the leading automobile manufacturing companies and developed in post World War II Japan, has been proposed as a model to address the concerns delineated in the *Future of Nursing* report.[8,9] As the Toyota Motor Company faced financial ruin, Skichi Toyoda led the development of the company's core philosophy and principles, which used a process-oriented systems model focusing on respect for people, teamwork, mutual trust and commitment, elimination of waste, and continuous quality improvement. In contrast to traditional hierarchical management structures, the TPS system valued the importance of partnerships between management and employees at all levels.[10]

The organizational hierarchy of the "Toyota Way" has been described by Liker as a pyramid of 4 key components, namely Philosophy, Process, People/Partners, and Problem Solving, with an emphasis on continuous improvement (*Kaizen* or good change) (**Fig. 1**).[10] Underlying these components are 14 Management Principles that have been operationalized in all aspects of TPS (**Table 1**).[11] The base of the pyramid, Philosophy, embodies the first of the 14 principles and underscores the importance of shared vision and long-term strategic thinking.[10] This principle promotes a shift from a quick-fix culture to a systems perspective based on a culture of long-term thinking, customer orientation, and cultural alignment of human and technical systems to support meaningful change.

The second tier of the pyramid, which focuses on efficient and effective production processes (reflecting TPS principles 2–8) is based on the belief that "the right process will produce the right results" and that every major innovation consists of several smaller prior innovations.[10,12] Within this tier, every failure and near miss within

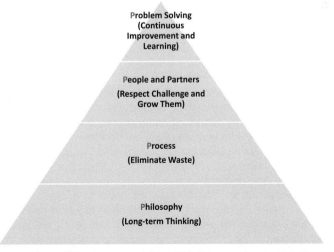

Fig. 1. The "4 P" model of the Toyota Production System. (*From* Liker JK. The Toyota Way: 14 principles from the world's greatest manufacturer. New York: McGraw Hill; 2004; with permission.)

Principle	Toyota Principle
Table 1 **The 14 principles of the Toyota Way**	
Section I: Long-Term Philosophy	
1	Base your management decisions on a long-term philosophy, even at the expense of short-term financial goals
Section II: The Right Process Will Produce the Right Results	
2	Create a continuous process flow to bring problems to the surface
3	Use "pull" systems to avoid overproduction
4	Level out the workload
5	Build a culture of stopping to fix problems, to get quality right the first time
6	Standardized tasks and processes are the foundation for continuous improvement and employee empowerment
7	Use visual control so no problems are hidden
8	Use only reliable, thoroughly tested technology that serves your people and processes
Section III: Add Value to the Organization by Developing Your People	
9	Grow leaders who thoroughly understand the work, live the philosophy, and teach it to others
10	Develop exceptional people and teams who follow your company's philosophy
11	Respect your extended network of partners and suppliers by challenging them and helping them improve
Section IV: Continuously Solving Root Problems Drives Organizational Learning	
12	Go and see for yourself to thoroughly understand the situation
13	Make decisions slowly by consensus, thoroughly considering all options; implement decisions rapidly
14	Become a learning organization through relentless reflection and continuous improvement

From Liker JK. The Toyota Way: 14 principles from the world's greatest manufacturer. New York: McGraw Hill; 2004; with permission.

organizational processes is studied from a systems perspective. Rather than placing "blame" on an individual, errors or defects are viewed as inadequate checks and balances within a system that should be designed to detect and neutralize mistakes before they occur. Within this systems perspective, all employees are expected and empowered to "stop the line" immediately if there is any deviation from established quality standards. Visual controls, which embody a unified team approach to quality standards, combined with a culture of transparency that celebrates identification and communication of defects in production, are core elements of the TPS model.

Within TPS, members of an organization are expected to critically examine process flow and bring both problems and inherent inefficiencies to the surface on an ongoing basis. Members are also committed to a lean production system, which results in enhanced operational efficiencies through an ongoing analysis of process flow, leveling of the workload, identification and elimination of waste and overproduction, and the effective use of human resources and technology. Organizational members focus on getting things right the first time, avoiding costly duplication and related risk. Standardization of tasks is also intended to support implementation of best practices and early identification of deviations in quality or process, so that immediate analysis and corrective action can be implemented.[10]

The third tier of the pyramid (TPS principles 9–11) emphasizes the value of people within the organization.[10] Recognizing that employees, partners, and stakeholders are the mind, heart, soul, and hands of TPS, executives, professional staff, and front-line production are considered equal partners in all aspects of daily work. Respect for individual contributions to the organization transcends occupational title or job description. There is an ongoing organizational commitment to attract and retain competent individuals, provide comprehensive education and training on an ongoing basis, and to grow leaders who thoroughly understand the work, live the philosophy, and teach it to others. Recruitment and retention activities include a system of shared incentives and rewards, formalized educational programs, on-the-job-training, and personal development opportunities. Human resource priorities are directed toward nurturing shared beliefs, engagement of employees who have a voice in the work of the organization, and fostering the development of employees who are committed to problem solving, continuous improvement, standardization of processes, and innovation, with the objectives of realizing company goals and benefiting both customers and employees.[13]

The highest level of the pyramid (TPS principles 12–14) focuses on respect, partnership, mutual trust, and commitment to continuous improvement within a learning organization.[10] Human and product value streams are inextricably intertwined with the belief that shared values, standardized processes, and the elimination of waste will produce the best results. Executives and front-line employees are considered equal partners on the workshop floor (*gemba*). Organizational members are encouraged to practice *Genchi-Genbutsu*, translated as going to the source to find the facts, making enlightened decisions, building consensus, and facilitating shared problem solving. *Genchi-Genbutsu* provides the foundation for a culture that supports stopping to fix problems and getting quality right the first time, for added value to customers and society.[12,13]

Leape[14] challenges that the current culture in health care is not only unsafe, but is dysfunctional as a result of: (1) an authoritarian culture that devalues workers; (2) a lack of personal accountability; (3) autonomous functioning in professional silos; and (4) major barriers to communication. Leape also contends that safety in health care cannot be achieved, no matter how many safe practices are implemented, without a change in organizational culture that values what everyone brings to the patient encounter as well as a dedication to a new systems-based model of education and practice.[14]

TOYOTA PRINCIPLES IN HEALTH CARE

In 2003, visionary leaders at Virginia Mason Medical Center (VMMC) in Seattle, Washington incorporated TPS throughout the organization in response to serious patient safety concerns and dwindling financial resources.[15] VMMC's Chief Executive Officer recognized the need for change and innovation. Through a chance meeting with a former airline executive, who introduced him to the successes achieved at Boeing and the application of TPS principles in the aviation industry, he embarked on a journey of revolutionizing patient care.[7,16] By 2010, after successful implementation of TPS throughout the organization, VMMC was a thriving medical institution that had saved $15 million in revenues over 6 years, and was named top hospital of the decade by the Leapfrog Group for improving the quality, safety, and affordability of health care.[17]

Other health care systems in Minnesota and Pennsylvania followed VMMC's example and enjoyed similar successes through TPS incorporation. In 2004, the Park Nicollet Medical Center in Minnesota, a leading health care institution, achieved

$7.5 million in savings using TPS.[18] In Pennsylvania, the Pittsburgh Veterans Administration Healthcare System reduced the incidence of hospital-acquired bacteria-resistant life-threatening infections in their surgical intensive care and surgical units by 82% through the incorporation of TPS.[19] The Lehigh Valley Health Network in eastern Pennsylvania, a Magnet designated organization, used TPS to reduce length of stay of patients, improve patient satisfaction, decrease emergency department diversions, and reduce time elapsed from patient admission to the emergency room to hospital bed.[20]

DREXEL UNIVERSITY'S JOURNEY

The Associate Dean of Nursing at Drexel University CNHP in Philadelphia appreciated the successes in patient safety outcomes achieved at these highly innovative health care organizations. She suggested that TPS might improve patient safety outcomes among nursing students during their clinical education. Moreover, she conjectured that TPS could facilitate the emergence of compassionate, culturally sensitive nursing graduates, who were adept at transdisciplinary collaboration, leadership, critical thinking, and lifelong learning as recommended by the RWJF-IOM Collaboration and the nursing student competency recommendations of the AACN.[2,21] Although an exhaustive literature search uncovered several research studies supporting successes in patient outcomes achieved through incorporation of TPS in clinical health care, the Associate Dean found a lack of published research examining patient outcomes and nursing student practices after incorporation of the TPS into nursing educational curricula.[22–25] She further recognized that the current state of nursing curricula was not positioned to facilitate the emergence of nursing graduates ready to meet society's increasing complex health care needs.

Nursing education has traditionally functioned within its own professional silo without affording nursing students the opportunity to practice transdisciplinary collaboration to decrease medical error and provide more efficient, quality patient care.[26] Historically, nursing curricula have been content-saturated and teacher-centered, promoting only superficial understanding of concepts.[27–29] Under this current educational system, nursing students often experience a combination of knowledge redundancy as well as significant gaps in other critical areas of learning. Within this system, students are often hesitant to reveal deficits in personal knowledge. Such an educational structure engenders error-prone individual problem solving, rather than group collaboration fostering safer patient care.

Clinical nursing education has also followed the same model, with very few exceptions. In this model clinical faculty assigns 8 to 10 students to a clinical area, where they both guide and evaluate learner outcomes. During each clinical rotation, student learning is often more centered on hospital or unit-specific orientation rather than on understanding the role and responsibilities of the professional nurse.[30] Furthermore, student success depends exclusively on the strengths of the individual clinical faculty member working with them in the clinical area.[31] This model of clinical education is losing relevance as changes in nursing practice are quickly shifting from antiquated methods that focus merely on acquisition of fundamental skills in favor of a community-based, transdisciplinary approach to patient care.[32,33]

Early Implementation

One of the first steps for implementation of TPS into Drexel University CNHP was a shift of administrative philosophy toward collaboration and transparency whereby faculty involvement was integral to incorporating TPS into the philosophy, culture, and the curriculum of the nursing undergraduate programs. As the Associate Dean of Drexel University CNHP was a Robert Wood Johnson (RWJ) Executive Nurse Fellow, she used RWJ funds to send a core group of nursing faculty to Seattle, Washington to develop an understanding of both the TPS model and how Virginia Mason translated the model to health care delivery. After the visit, the core nursing faculty returned convinced that many of the same tenets applied to clinical practice within the hospital environment were also relevant to nursing education. The core group envisioned incorporating the same safety practices and TPS into the nursing curriculum to promote a culture of safety among students that would continue into their future roles in professional practice.

The core faculty shared their knowledge gained from the VMMC visit with the remainder of the faculty, and TPS incorporation was fully vetted in the undergraduate nursing curriculum committee. Drexel nursing faculty serving as course chairs then worked with their respective course faculty to explore opportunities to operationalize the Toyota principles as applicable to their respective courses. The information was also disseminated to clinical faculty in course-specific orientation sessions and in quarterly adjunct faculty educational seminars. The principle of going to the *gemba* was put to use through conscious efforts to enhance problem identification and collaborative problem solving among full-time faculty, clinical adjunct faculty, and students and staff at all levels both in the classroom and in clinical settings, exemplifying TPS principles 12, 13, and 14. As a result, several modifications were made to the nursing curriculum and pedagogy based on adaptation of the TPS principles and practices.

Although VMMC pioneered TPS in the health care setting, Drexel University CNHP is the first academic institution to introduce it into nursing education. In 2011, the school revised its curriculum to incorporate pertinent TPS principles with a focus on quality and safety. In September 2011, the program was officially rolled out to students and integrated throughout the curriculum. Consistent with the third tier of the TPS, which emphasizes the value of people within the organization and provision of opportunities for personal and professional development, educational forums were used to translate TPS principles into nursing education among both students and faculty within the classroom and clinical settings.[12]

Classroom Incorporation of TPS

Consistent with the beliefs that early immersion into the culture of safety and development of a sense of personal and professional accountability in all students was a fundamental element, a new course emphasizing TPS principles was introduced during the first quarter of nursing classes. The format of this new course included both lecture content and application of theory in group-learning activities and discussions. A highly interactive classroom environment emphasized collaboration and sharing of ideas within a problem-based learning model.

According to the report from the IOM, *To Err is Human*, the most common cause for medical errors is miscommunication among health care providers.[5] Furthermore, nursing students as well as experienced nurses are often hesitant to voice concerns about patient care to physicians.[34–36] In response to these issues, students at Drexel University CNHP are taught to use a standardized tool to communicate critical patient information with other caregivers. SBAR (Situation, Background, Assessment, and Recommendation) is a tool recommended by the IHI for the purpose of improving the effectiveness of communication among caregivers.[37] It is based on similar communication tools used in the aviation industry. This technique represents a hybrid of medical and nursing communication styles intended to enhance nurse-physician communication. Kesten[38] discovered that students who learned SBAR by both didactic instruction and role play performed significantly better than those who learned solely by didactic instruction.

Students are initially taught SBAR communication in the classroom, whereas reinforcement and further learning takes place through situational role play and clinical simulations. Aled[39] demonstrated that knowledge from the classroom is not always effortlessly transferred to the clinical area. Therefore, it is best to afford students opportunities to learn and apply theoretical principles of nursing care in a safe simulation environment away from the bedside.[40]

Teaching students to voice concerns is also reinforced in Drexel's Nursing Leadership course. Simulations, enacted and video-recorded in the simulation laboratory, are then broadcast into the classroom. One such simulation involves an impaired nurse, novice nurse, and nurse manager. The impaired nurse is suspected of diverting opiates, and bullies the novice nurse (played by a student) by asking the novice nurse to sign-out the drug for her. Following the presentation, students discuss the scenario and faculty provides debriefing. Feedback from students suggests that this experience has helped them to learn how to handle real situations they might encounter as a professional nurse. This simulation experience has also assisted them in learning how to be assertive with another health care provider and nurse manager so as to avoid nonprofessional nursing practice and potential errors in patient care. Through this simulation experience, students have learned to stop and fix problems so that a culture of safety can be maintained. The essential features for this particular scenario are the visual and verbal cues presented by the impaired nurse, so students can be directed to learn the signs of possible on-the-job substance abuse (TPS principles 3, 5, 7, 9, and 10).[11]

Incorporation of Active Learning Strategies

In an effort to provide student-centered learning, Drexel faculty has enlisted a variety of active learning strategies. Cooperative learning is one such activity whereby small teams of students work together to improve their understanding of a topic. Each team member is responsible for their own learning as well as learning of the other students within their team. Group members then critique one another's contributions and leadership of the group.[41]

Other types of active learning strategies used by Drexel University CNHP faculty include concept mapping, problem-based learning, role play, and unfolding case studies. Each of these strategies is a nontraditional method of instruction whereby students are moved to the role of decision maker. Faculty guides students to resources and information necessary to formulate questions, explore alternatives, and make decisions. Because situations must be realistic and believable to students, learning materials must be designed to bring real-world problems into the classroom for open exploration. Findings from prior research suggest that these learning strategies directly enhance critical thinking and communication between students and faculty, exemplifying TPS principles 13 and 14.[42]

Clinical Incorporation of TPS

Using the TPS system, Drexel University CNHP nursing students caring for patients in the clinical area are taught a variety of approaches to help assure patient safety. Based on the knowledge that the right processes will produce the right results, students begin their clinical day by learning to use a 1-minute checklist to identify any pertinent safety issues, exemplifying TPS principles 3, 5, 6, and 7, analogous to the pilot of a airplane who makes a series of checks before taking off. Gawande,[43] who instituted the use of checklists in medicine while working with the World Health Organization, found that checklists could be useful in promoting patient safety.

Before TPS incorporation, Drexel University CNHP faculty supervised student medication administration in the clinical area by instructing students to pull each medication from the medication cart as they explained its indications, actions, side effects, and special nursing precautions. Students stated anecdotally that they felt distracted by this practice. According to recent nursing research, the 2 most common factors contributing to medication errors were interruption and distractions during administration.[44–47] Based on student input, review of the literature, and TPS principles 3 and 6, this method of instruction was abandoned. Faculty now ensures minimal distraction and interruption while nursing students pour and administer medications to patients.

Miscalculation of medication dosage also remains one of the most frequent mistakes made by nursing students.[48] These errors may result in part from student confusion that ensues after learning multiple methods of dosage calculation from a variety of faculty and tutors.[49,50] In addition, some of these ineffective methods are based on tradition rather than evidence-based practice. TPS principle 6 encompasses the value of standardization to prevent error. Standardization is based on capturing the accumulated learning about a process up to a point in time by standardizing best practices. To reduce student error, the Drexel team adopted standardized medication dosage calculation through the use of dimensional analysis to calculate drug dosages instead of ratio-proportion and/or formula methods.[51–53] Dimensional analysis, also known as the factor-label method, conversion-factor method, units analysis, and quantity calculus, provides a systematic way to set up problems, and assists students in organizing and evaluating data.[54] This method involves the logical sequencing and placement into an equation of all of the arithmetical terms (both quantities and units) involved in the problems such that all of the units cancel out except the unit(s) of the desired answer (eg, milligrams, drops per minute).

As Drexel University CNHP continued the process of standardization, faculty also improved techniques for teaching and testing nursing skills and physical assessment in the clinical laboratory as well as the clinical area. Before this change, students often expressed confusion in learning these skills because the learning techniques changed as they moved from course to course. Students began to use electronic forms with step-by-step standardized procedures housed in an online software package (Waypoint).[55] This method provided a mechanism whereby faculty could enter comments alongside student scores at the site of testing to provide immediate feedback. By standardizing techniques for teaching physical assessment and nursing skills, students experienced less confusion through elimination of variance in faculty teaching methods.

Low-fidelity and high-fidelity simulations are offered throughout Drexel University CNHP clinical curriculum. In the foundational nursing practice course, students participate in 4 different situational assessments. Students are given 60 seconds from the time they enter a patient room setup in the clinical laboratory to "notice" any inherent errors or problems. Through observation, students learn the art of vigilance and use SBAR while communicating their findings to laboratory faculty.[56] Ebright and colleagues[57] describe vigilance as an "intentional and knowledgeable watchfulness of the patient, the care environment, and one's own thinking."

As students move through the nursing program, communication aptitude is expected to further develop. Thus activities are built into the clinical curriculum that calls for students to work in intradisciplinary and transdisciplinary work groups. The standardized patient experience is used in several courses so that students learn to sharpen their communication skills with patients and family members. Interdisciplinary clinical work provides the opportunity to develop communication and clinical decision-making skills in scenarios involving registered nurses in the roles of professional colleague, nurse manager, and nurse practitioner.

Although rapid response teams have been instituted to prevent adverse hospital events leading to disability and death, each year many preventable deaths occur in acute care facilities. These events may result from the failure of the health care team to quickly respond to patients exhibiting signs and symptoms of impending distress. Such events have been termed "failure to rescue" and claim at least 61,000 lives annually.[58] Within Drexel University CNHP, senior nursing students are exposed to failure-to-rescue scenarios within interdisciplinary simulation experiences in their capstone course. The purpose of these high-fidelity cases is to familiarize students with real-life situations, which require them to recognize patient decompensation trends and intervene appropriately. Faculty agrees that additional student competencies necessary for success are teamwork and effective communication, exemplifying TPS principles 3, 5, and 7.[11]

Drexel faculty also developed a transdisciplinary simulation aimed at breaking down the professional silos within health care. The simulation involved women's health care student providers including undergraduate nursing students, nurse practitioner students, medical students, obstetrics and gynecology residents, nurse anesthetist students, and physician assistant students. A scenario based on emergency management of unanticipated shoulder dystocia and postpartum hemorrhage in a 25-year-old woman, who had inadequate prenatal care, was presented to the group. Students were expected to work together as a team to care for mother and infant. The Team Strategies and Tools to Enhance Performance and Patient Safety, " an evidence-based teamwork system to improve communication and teamwork skills among health care professionals" developed jointly by the AHRQ and the Department of Defense, provided the conceptual framework for this experience.[59] The various types of simulations exemplified TPS principles 3, 4, 5, 6, 7, 9, 10, 11, and 14.

Toyota principle 8 emphasizes the use of "reliable, thoroughly tested technology that serves people and processes."[12] Drexel faculty educates students to use an electronic medical record to practice patient information retrieval and documentation. Students are taught to be facile in obtaining information from their iPod Touch device while in the clinical learning center, simulation laboratory, and during standardized patient experiences. More than 2500 medical applications (apps) are available from the iTunes store with 300 directly related to nursing.[60] Clinical resources from an electronic library of textbooks loaded onto iPods are available to students to access information at the point of patient care. Williams and Dittmer[61] found that e-books provide students with increased speed and retrieval of evidence-based information at the bedside. In this study, students experienced increased confidence in the clinical setting as well as reduced time needed for clinical preparation.

RECOMMENDATIONS (LOOKING BACK...MOVING FORWARD)

Initial efforts of translating the TPS model into the nursing curriculum have already made a significant impact on the context and process of curricular revision in Drexel's nursing program. However, in retrospect Drexel faculty realizes that initial incorporation efforts were grounded in a quick-fix results orientation focusing on integration of Quality and Safety Education for Nurses and other safety standards into the nursing curriculum, without significant emphasis on developing a grassroots understanding and faculty enculturation into the Toyota philosophy. Lack of attention to generating consensus about initial implementation was quickly overcome, however, as faculty embraced a commitment to emphasize safety in all aspects of the undergraduate nursing program. Once that common goal was realized, the necessary cultural shift began to emerge naturally.

Feedback from Drexel's health care partners and varied stakeholder groups suggested the need for increased emphasis on leadership development, communication skills, critical thinking and problem-solving skills, and effective team interactions in the nursing curriculum. Consistent with the belief that high standards and efficient systems will produce high-quality results, Drexel's emphasis has shifted from an initial quick-fix orientation on quality standards to a "process," people-oriented focus for curriculum revision embodying long-term thinking, efficient and effective systems, technology as added value, and teamwork within an environment committed to quality outcomes and continuous improvement.

While significant progress has been made in a relatively short time, there is still much to be done to firmly incorporate the tenets of the TPS model into Drexel's nursing program philosophy and practice. The DNA of Toyota lies in its culture.[12] Drexel faculty now understands the need to incorporate TPS as an interconnected whole woven into the philosophy and mission of the nursing program beyond the isolated focus of curriculum reform. The emphasis now is to build on the work of early adopters and grow leaders among faculty, students, and graduates who understand the work of nursing education and practice, live the philosophy, and can teach it to others. It is recognized that TPS must evolve into a system of thinking whereby the varied stakeholders can have input into both the process and outcomes of the nursing educational experience.

Lack of shared philosophy and vision will facilitate programmatic failure rather than success within the educational institution.[10,11,13,62] The systems perspective of quality at the point of care has begun to narrow the gap between education and practice and has created opportunities for enhanced collaboration, cooperation, and dialogue with health care providers, educators, and employers, which has resulted in enhanced learning opportunities for students and will continue to provide valuable insight for ongoing curricular revisions for the foreseeable future.

SUMMARY

The TPS model has enjoyed success in promoting excellence in both industry and health care settings. This article describes the first known attempt at applying TPS principles in nursing education. The experience and results of this initiative suggest that the philosophy, principles, and practices inherent in the TPS system can be easily adapted and can provide a foundation to address contemporary challenges in nursing education. With established credibility in both industry and health care settings, TPS also provides a common ground and language that will serve as a basis to bridge the gap between education and practice.

Further exploration of the TPS and lessons learned from industry cannot be overlooked by nursing educators in an effort to develop meaningful curricular reform that will serve students and health care providers, and have a positive impact on the delivery of health care services to the public. Experiences in industry and health care facilities, such as Virginia Mason and others, have suggested that valuing, nurturing, and empowering individuals who are committed to organizational goals, cost-effective and cost-efficient production systems, and high-quality outcomes can produce superior results. Continued exploration of the TPS model as an element of curricular reform, combined with collaboration, research, and widespread dissemination of findings and experiences will serve to enhance understanding and promote meaningful curricular innovation, and serve as a basis for ongoing advancement of contemporary nursing education and practice.

ACKNOWLEDGMENTS

The authors wish to thank Dr Mary Ellen Smith Glasgow, Former Associate Dean for Nursing at Drexel University College of Nursing and Health Professions for her leadership on this project and the Robert Wood Johnson Foundation for funding faculty attendance at the Virginia Mason Institute.

REFERENCES

1. Patient Care and Affordable Care Act, 2010: United States.
2. Institute of Medicine. The future of nursing: leading change, advancing health. 2010. Available at: http://www.iom.edu/Reports/2010/The-Future-of-Nursing-Leading-Change-Advancing-Health.aspx. Accessed April 17, 2012.
3. American Association of Colleges of Nursing. Competency report from the IPEC panel. In: Team-Based Competencies, editor. Building a shared foundation for education and clinical practice. Washington, DC: Robert Wood Johnson Foundation; 2011. p. 1–24.
4. Institute of Medicine. Crossing the quality chasm: a new health system for the 21st century. 2001. Available at: http://iom.edu/Reports/2001/Crossing-the-Quality-Chasm-A-New-Health-System-for-the-21st-Century.aspx. Accessed April 17, 2012.
5. Institute of Medicine. To err is human: building a safer health system. 2000. Available at: http://www.nap.edu/openbook.php?isbn=0309068371. Accessed April 17, 2012.
6. Leape LL, Berwick DM, Bates DW. What practices will most improve safety? JAMA 2002;288(4):501–7.
7. Kenney C. Transforming health care: Virginia Mason Medical Center's pursuit of the perfect patient experience. New York: CRC Press; 2011.
8. Campbell RJ, Gantt L, Congdon T. Teaching workflow analysis and lean thinking via simulation: a formative evaluation. Perspect Health Inf Manag 2009;6:3.
9. Thompson DN, Wolf GA, Spear SJ. Driving improvement in patient care: lessons from Toyota. J Nurs Adm 2003;33(11):585–95.
10. Liker JK. The Toyota Way: 14 principles from the world's greatest manufacturer. New York: McGraw Hill; 2004.
11. Liker JK, Meier M. The Toyota Way fieldbook: a practical guide for implementing Toyota's 4Ps. New York: McGraw Hill; 2006.
12. Liker JK, Hoseus M. Toyota culture: the heart and soul of the Toyota way. New York: McGraw Hill; 2008.
13. Liker JK, Meier M. Toyota talent: developing your people the Toyota way. New York: McGraw Hill; 2007.
14. Leape LL. Errors in medicine. Clin Chim Acta 2009;404(1):2–5.
15. Ziskovsky B, Ziskovsky J. Doing more with less—going lean in education: a white paper on process improvement in education. 2007. Available at: http://www.leaneducation.com/whitepaper/whitepaper-DoingMoreWithLess.pdf. Accessed April 10, 2010.
16. Blackmore CC, Mecklenburg RS, Kaplan GS. At Virginia Mason, collaboration among providers, employers, and health plans to transform care cut costs and improved quality. Health Aff 2011;30(9):1680–7.
17. Group L. The Leapfrog Group announces top hospitals of the decade. 2010. Available at: http://www.leapfroggroup.org/news/leapfrog_news/4784721. Accessed April 17, 2012.
18. Varkey P, Reller MK, Resar RK. Basics of quality improvement in health care. Mayo Clin Proc 2007;82(6):735–9.

19. Richmond I, et al. Best-practice protocols: reducing harm from MRSA. Nurs Manag 2007;38(8):22–7.
20. Korner KT, Hartman NM, Agee A, et al. Lean tools and concepts reduce waste, improve efficiency. Am Nurse Today 2011;6(3):41–4.
21. American Association of Colleges of Nursing. The essentials of baccalaureate education from nursing practice. 2012. Available at: http://www.aacn.nche.edu/Education/pdf/BaccEssentials08.pdf. Accessed April 17, 2012.
22. Culig MH, et al. Improving patient care in cardiac surgery using Toyota production system based methodology. Ann Thorac Surg 2011;91(2):394–9.
23. Furman C, Caplan R. Applying the Toyota production system: using a patient safety alert system to reduce error. Joint Comm J Qual Patient Saf 2007;33(7):376–86.
24. Newell TL, Steinmetz-Malato LL, Van Dyke DL. Applying Toyota production system techniques for medication delivery: improving hospital safety and efficiency. J Healthc Qual 2011;33(2):115–22.
25. Young JQ, Wachter RM. Applying Toyota production system principles to a psychiatric hospital: making transfers safer and more timely. Joint Comm J Qual Patient Saf 2009;35(9):439–48.
26. Ironside PM, Sitterding M. Embedding quality and safety competencies in nursing education. J Nurs Educ 2009;48(12):659–60.
27. Jeffries PR, Rew S, Cramer JM. A comparison of student-centered versus traditional methods of teaching basic nursing skills in a learning laboratory. Nurs Educ Perspect 2002;23(1):14–9.
28. Giddens JF, Brady DP. Rescuing nursing education from content saturation: the case for a concept-based curriculum. J Nurs Educ 2007;46(2):65–9.
29. Candela L, Dalley K, Benzel-Lindley J. A case for learning-centered curricula. J Nurs Educ 2006;45(2):59–66.
30. MacIntyre RC, et al. Common themes in clinical education partnerships. J Nurs Educ 2011;50(7):366–72.
31. MacIntyre RC, et al. Five recommendations for prelicensure clinical nursing education. J Nurs Educ 2009;48(8):447–53.
32. Tanner CA. Transforming prelicensure nursing education: preparing the new nurse to meet emerging health care needs. Nurs Educ Perspect 2010;31(6):347–53.
33. Porter-O'Grady T, Afable R. Reforming the healthcare structure. Health Prog 2002;83(1):17–20.
34. Lawrence KM, et al. Perceived information needs and communication difficulties of inpatient physicians and nurses. J Am Med Inform Assoc 2002;9(6):S64–9.
35. McCaffrey RG, et al. A program to improve communication and collaboration between nurses and medical residents. J Contin Educ Nurs 2010;41(4):172–8.
36. Myers S, et al. Safety concerns of hospital-based new-to-practice registered nurses and their preceptors. J Contin Educ Nurs 2010;41(4):163–71.
37. Staff KP. SBAR: situation-background-assessment-recommendation. 2012. Available at: http://www.ihi.org/explore/SBARCommunicationTechnique/Pages/default.aspx. Accessed April 22, 2012.
38. Kesten KS. Role-play using SBAR technique to improve observed communication skills in senior nursing students. J Nurs Educ 2011;50(2):79–87.
39. Aled J. Putting practice into teaching: an exploratory study of nursing undergraduates' interpersonal skills and the effects of using empirical data as a teaching and learning resource. J Clin Nurs 2007;16:2297–307.
40. Bambini D, Washburn J, Perkins R. Outcomes of clinical simulation for novice nursing students: communication, confidence, clinical judgment. Nurs Educ Perspect 2009;30(2):79–82.

41. Stiles AS. Cooperative learning: enhancing individual learning through positive group process. Annu Rev Nurs Educ 2006;4:131–59.
42. Joel LA. Instructional methods. In: Moyer BA, Wittmann-Price RA, editors. Nursing education: foundations for practice excellence. Philadelphia: F. A. Davis; 2008. p. 183–211.
43. Gawande A. The checklist manifesto: how to get things right. New York: Metropolitan Books; 2009.
44. Biron AD, Lavoie-Tremblay M, Loiselle CG. Characteristics of work interruptions during medication administration. J Nurs Scholarsh 2009;41(4):330–6.
45. Nguyen EE, Connolly PM, Wong V. Medication safety initiative in reducing medication errors. J Nurs Care Qual 2010;25(3):224–30.
46. Pape TM, et al. Innovative approaches to reducing nurses' distractions during medication administration. J Contin Educ Nurs 2005;36(3):108–16 [quiz: 141–2].
47. Trbovich P, et al. Interruptions during the delivery of high-risk medications. J Nurs Adm 2010;40(5):211–8.
48. Wolf ZR, Hicks R, Serembus JF. Characteristics of medication errors made by students during the administration phase: a descriptive study. J Prof Nurs 2006;22(1):39–51.
49. Dexter P, Applegate M. How to solve a math problem. J Nurs Educ 1980;19(2): 49–53.
50. Worrell PJ, Hodson KE. Posology: the battle against dosage calculation errors. Nurse Educ 1989;14(2):27–31.
51. Greenfield S, Whelan B, Cohn E. Use of dimensional analysis to reduce medication errors. J Nurs Educ 2006;45(2):91–4.
52. Rice JN, Bell ML. Using dimensional analysis to improve drug dosage calculation ability. J Nurs Educ 2005;44(7):315–8.
53. Serembus JF. Medication calculation ability of baccalaureate nursing students as a function of method of instruction, in DAI. Philadelphia: Widener; 2000.
54. Craig GP. Clinical calculations made easy: solving problems using dimensional analysis. 5th edition. Philadelphia: Lippincott; 2011.
55. Schlitz SA, et al. Developing a culture of assessment through a faculty learning community: a case study. IJTLHE 2006;21(1):133–47.
56. Struth D, et al. The 60 second situational assessment. 2009. Available at: http://www.qsen.org/teachingstrategy.php?id=89. Accessed April 17, 2012.
57. Ebright PR, et al. Mindful attention to complexity: implications for teaching and learning patient safety in nursing. Annu Rev Nurs Educ 2006;4:339–60.
58. Reed K, et al. HealthGrades sixth annual patient safety in American Hospitals Study. 2009. Available at: http://www.healthgrades.com/business/img/PatientSafetyInAmericanHospitalsStudy2009.pdf. Accessed April 17, 2012.
59. AHRQ. TeamSTEPPS® fundamentals course: Module 1. Evidence-base: introduction/team structure. 2010. Available at: http://www.ahrq.gov/teamsteppstools/instructor/fundamentals/module1/m1evidencebase.htm. Accessed April 22, 2012.
60. Skiba DJ. Back to school: what's in your students' backpacks? Nurs Educ Perspect 2010;31(5):318–20.
61. Williams MG, Dittmer A. Textbooks on tap: using electronic books housed in handheld devices in nursing clinical courses. Nurs Educ Perspect 2009;30(4): 220–5.
62. Ballé M, Régnier A. Lean as a learning system in a hospital ward. Leader Health Serv 2007;20(1):33–41.

Preparing Nurses to Care for People with Developmental Disabilities

Perspectives on Integrating Developmental Disabilities Concepts and Experiences into Nursing Education

Marcia R. Gardner, PhD, RN, CPNP, CPN

KEYWORDS

- Autism • Intellectual and developmental disabilities • Nursing education

KEY POINTS

- Nurses in all settings and specialties will encounter increasing numbers of patients with developmental disabilities (DDs).
- Nursing curricula should address concepts of care for people with DDs across the life span and should develop strategies to provide students with clinically relevant experiences to develop care competencies for this population.
- Exemplar strategies from the literature are described along with recommendations for further work.

INTRODUCTION

Developmental disabilities (DDs), according to the federal Developmental Disabilities Bill of Rights Act (2000),[1] are chronic conditions that develop before age 22 that result in significantly impaired cognitive and/or physical functioning in at least 3 domains of life, persist long term or throughout the life span, and result in prolonged or lifelong need for services, support, or assistance. Communication, mobility, learning, self-direction, and independent living may be affected. DD is an umbrella concept under which many conditions, such as cerebral palsy, autism, and intellectual disabilities, can be clustered, depending on the degree and pervasiveness of functional and cognitive impairment, per the federal definition. Although they are different, there is overlap among characteristics associated with intellectual disability and developmental disability. For brevity, this term, DDs, is used in this article to include all or any of these

Disclosures: The author does not have a relationship with a commercial company that has a direct financial interest in the subject matter or materials discussed in this article.
Department of Family Nursing, College of Nursing, Seton Hall University, 400 South Orange Avenue, NJ 973-761-9295, USA
E-mail address: Marcia.Gardner@shu.edu

Nurs Clin N Am 47 (2012) 517–527
http://dx.doi.org/10.1016/j.cnur.2012.07.010
0029-6465/12/$ – see front matter © 2012 Elsevier Inc. All rights reserved.

conditions across the life span. The population of individuals with DDs is diverse, with diverse and wide-ranging capabilities and health care needs.

Nurses in practice report that their educational preparation to care for this population is inadequate. They experience difficulties caring for patients with communication, social, cognitive, behavioral, physical, and other challenges associated with many of these conditions in many health care settings.[2–4] Hahn[3] has argued for better education of nurses about DDs, emphasizing both preparation for entry into practice and continuing education. Now, this gap is of even more concern and growing urgency, considering the large number of children being diagnosed with DDs, such as autism, both in the United States and around the globe.[5–7] Acute care, primary care, long-term care, and community, school health, and support services for individuals with DDs and their families will be increasingly needed as children with DDs become adults and older adults and as their caregivers age as well.[8] Nurses will be challenged to integrate the rapidly growing body of evidence related to causes and interventions for people with DDs into their practice and to provide the most appropriate and effective, yet cost-effective, care.

SIGNIFICANCE: POPULATION CONSIDERATIONS

Both federal and state laws define DDs for funding and service provision purposes. State-level DDs services and their criteria vary, especially those for adults with developmental conditions.[9] Mechanisms for collecting information about the populations involved also vary by state, and accurate national population data, especially on adults, are difficult to obtain.[10] Recent studies of children indicate, however, that the size of the population of people with DDs across the life span is increasing. This is most likely associated with the growing numbers of children diagnosed with conditions that fall under the DDs umbrella, in particular autism.[5,11] In the adult noninstitutionalized population, the prevalence of DDs between 1994 and 1995 was estimated at 14.9 per 1000 individuals.[12] There is also a growing group of aging adults with DDs who will most likely require specialized health care services in specialized settings that accommodate their needs as older adults and as individuals with DDs.[13]

Between 1997–1999 and 2006–2008, the prevalence of DDs in children increased 17.1%, whereas the prevalence of autism spectrum disorders grew by an astounding 289.5%.[5–7] The prevalence of DDs was estimated to be 1:6 children between 3 and 17 years of age in 2008.[5] The most recent estimate of the prevalence of autism spectrum disorders in the United States was reported to be 1:88 children (8 years of age).[14] The increased prevalence of DDs in children is believed related to several factors. These include survival of extremely low birth weight, extremely premature infants whose gestational status places them at risk for overt and subtle neurologic impairment and DDs, improved medical care of infants and children with neurologic and/or other physical disorders, and increased vigilance in screening for autism and developmental risks in general.[5]

The significance of these data is obvious: (1) there are more individuals with DD-related diagnoses and labels; (2) the growing population of children experiencing DDs will become a population of adults and older adults; (3) these individuals will need safe and high-quality health services provided by nurses with the necessary knowledge, skills, values, and ethical grounding to promote positive health care outcomes; (4) nurses in health care, home, and community settings of all sorts will most likely encounter individuals with DDs who will require their services integrated within a team approach to care; (5) nursing education programs at both prelicensure and graduate levels will need to better equip graduates with the competencies for appropriate care for this population of people; and (6) preparation of nurses to care for individuals with autism in particular is of increasing importance because this population has grown rapidly.

Although practicing clinicians may specialize and/or become certified in intellectual disabilities/DDs nursing,[15–17] most nurses and health care professionals are not specialists in this area and most do not practice in specialized developmental settings.[18] Yet most or all will encounter patients with DDs, regardless of clinical setting or their particular clinical specialties. A greater emphasis on preparing those who provide care for individuals with DDs in the health care system, across all specialties and all settings, is crucial. Nursing curricula at all levels should help students master the essential competencies to provide optimal care for the population of people with DDs. Nurses in all settings should feel, and be, well prepared by their educational programs to recognize condition-specific health risks in this population in order to be effective advocates for their patients or clients and families and to use best practice approaches in the management of health needs and those of families and caregivers.

To ensure that students develop basic competencies for the care of people with DD, they need to be assisted to create a toolkit of knowledge and skills and should have clinical involvement with the population. Such a toolkit can be thought of as knowledge of DDs legal guidelines related to people with disabilities, risks and precipitating factors (eg, genetics), associated health problems and related care and treatment, and assessment, decision-making, ethical reasoning, and case-finding skills; ability to apply developmental processes in context; family and individual collaboration skills; support and referral skills; and communication, interaction, and, importantly, strategies to effectively work with individuals who may exhibit challenging, disruptive, or atypical behaviors; have cognitive, social, and/or communication challenges; and/or are differently motivated. As with other populations of individuals with complex health needs, care of those with DDs also requires an effective interdisciplinary team approach, effective case management, and a health care home.[19] Students' mastery of competencies related to such components of safe, quality health care can be facilitated through curricular integration of relevant information, practice in clinical decision-making, and meaningful clinical experiences with people with DDs and with the health care team, in a variety of clinical settings—that is, in the settings where students will encounter and care for this population.

Both graduate and undergraduate curricula are important to consider. Smeltzer and colleagues[20] surveyed 234 undergraduate nursing programs and reported that most prelicensure nursing curricula included some information about disabilities in general and approximately 79% had information about DDs/intellectual disabilities specifically. Little is known about depth, proportion of time in the curriculum, and type of information or about clinical exposure to patients with these conditions. Most content related to DDs is placed in nursing of children, community, or psychiatric nursing courses in prelicensure curricula,[3,20] although clinicians care for patients with DDs in multiple settings and specialties.[2,16,17]

Nehring emphasized the need to expand the cadre of specialists in DDs nursing via graduate education and highlighted the advanced practice nursing (APN) curricula and federal training programs, such as Leadership Education in Neurodevelopmental Disabilities, which prepare specialists. These provide opportunities for students to refine knowledge and skills related to the assessment and care of developmentally vulnerable or developmentally disabled individuals and their families and to develop leadership skills as well as skills for practice as members of an interdisciplinary team.[16,17,21] Considering that individuals with DDs also need to access primary, acute, long-term care and community, hospice, and multiple other health services where DD nursing specialists may not be available, however, more general competencies for their care need to also be carefully addressed in graduate nursing education. There is sparse information in the literature about the actual level and extent of DDs content and clinical exposure to patients with DDs in APN nursing preparation, such as those programs preparing primary care nurse practitioners, clinical nurse specialists, nurse anesthetists, acute care nurse practitioners, and nurse midwives. Although Melnyk and colleagues[22] described curricular improvements in pediatric APN programs related to developmental, mental, and behavioral problems, the extent of integration of such content and, specifically, DDs or intellectual disabilities content in programs preparing APNs for family and adult care is not well described. APNs in primary care and other settings need to be equally well prepared to care for this growing population of individuals.

EDUCATION OF HEALTH CARE PROVIDERS TO ADDRESS GAPS AND DISPARITIES

Gaps in health care providers' knowledge and skills along with negative attitudes about individuals with disabilities and DDs are well known barriers to their access to high quality health care.[23–25] These concerns are not limited to the United States but have been echoed in the nursing literature from Australia, New Zealand, Greece, and Canada, and other countries.[26–30] Individuals with DDs or intellectual disabilities historically have been subject to stigmatization, marginalization, and paternalism in the health care system and to unsupported assumptions by health care clinicians about their behaviors, capabilities, and needs, and perceptions about their quality of life.[31]

Children who have DDs, especially those with associated behavioral disorders, often have complex associated conditions and multiple special health care needs, which require multidisciplinary involvement and frequent visits to health care providers, specialists, and acute care facilities[32] where nurses and APNs are involved in their care. Families of children with DDs report that they experience barriers to accessing appropriate care (ie, inappropriate or absent referrals and lack of access to appropriately prepared clinicians), poor communication among clinicians and family members, and cultural dissonance. They believe that clinicians are not well prepared to meet the specialized needs of children with DDs and report unmet health and family support needs.[10,33,34] They further report concerns about clinicians' knowledge of developmental disorders, understanding of their children's and adult children's behaviors, and competencies to deal with both behavior and other health problems related to the particular conditions as well as concerns about clinicians' competencies to deal with health problems and behaviors.[23]

Smeltzer and colleagues[35] reported similar themes in a qualitative study of adults with disabilities. Their sample included individuals with different disabilities, including those are categorized as DDs. They reported that concerns about communication, competence of nurses, negative attitudes, and care quality were major themes from the data. Adults with DD-related conditions have significantly poorer health than adults in the general population and have more difficulty accessing and using health services of all kinds. They are also less likely than other adults to receive health promotion-focused and preventive care and to engage in health promotion self-care activities, with associated increased risks for chronic illness and complications.[36]

Studies of nurses in practice found that they recall little exposure to information about intellectual disabilities and DDs and little to no clinical involvement with individuals with such conditions in their nursing education programs. They may demonstrate negative attitudes toward patients with these conditions.[2,24,37] Individuals with atypical or disruptive behaviors and limited communication skills, such as people with autism, may be particularly challenging for nurses to care for. People with autism spectrum disorders can be perceived as more difficult to care for than other individuals[38] and are likely perceived as even more so in the clinical setting due to unfamiliar staff and routines, fatigue, discomfort, or pain related to illness and treatment and the fast pace of care.

Specialized nursing strategies are often required to provide even basic health care services to people with autism.[4,39] Clearly health care education is falling short in preparing clinicians for best practice care of individuals with DD, and their families.

FACULTY CONSIDERATIONS

Smeltzer and colleagues[20,40] discussed the urgent need to enhance the nursing curricular focus on life span physical disabilities, mental disabilities, and DDs. They further documented gaps and variations in undergraduate nursing curricula and undergraduate nursing texts related to health care of the population of disabled individuals. According to Smeltzer and colleagues,[40] texts and curricular approaches, written or designed by nurses, continue to emphasize *dis*-ability in patients and to emphasize a paternalistic medical or rehabilitative perspective in nursing care. Smeltzer and colleagues[20] also noted that it is important for students and faculty to understand the strengths and the limitations of such models and to consider alternative philosophies and models of care that promote autonomy and that acknowledge and capitalize on individual, family, and community strengths. An initial study suggests that nursing faculty, like nurses as a group, have negative attitudes about people with disabilities in general,[41] but information about nursing faculty attitudes toward and knowledge about individuals with DDs in particular is limited. Despite this evidence gap, it is not a huge leap of logic to hypothesize that some nursing faculty members have less than optimal knowledge and skills for the care of individuals with disabilities in general and for the care of those with DDs in particular, perhaps associated with less than optimal preparation in their own programs of study and limited experience with the population in clinical practice. More exploration of faculty perceptions and competencies for care of individuals with DD is needed. Smeltzer and colleagues reported that faculty expertise in care of people with disabilities facilitated integration of such content in undergraduate curricula; they emphasized the need for continuing education for faculty to promote the development of such expertise.

Computer-based and web-based programs and modules for basic and continuing education in care of individuals with intellectual disabilities and DDs have been developed and are increasingly available for faculty and student use.[3,16,17] Giarelli and colleagues[42] developed a continuing education course specifically to educate nurses about autism. Educational programs of this nature address knowledge and attitudes,[3,43] but it is not clear if these are the best approach to prepare faculty to mentor students in the care of this population in the clinical setting, where in real time, assumptions and attitudes interact unpredictably with knowledge, skills, and theory. Experience with individuals who have various disabilities has been reported associated with more positive clinician, student, and nurse educator attitudes about them.[41,44,45] This phenomenon needs examination in the context of DDs.

INCORPORATION OF DD CONCEPTS AND EXPERIENCES IN NURSING EDUCATION

Nursing curricula at all levels, in one way or another, require mastery of discipline-specific and interdisciplinary knowledge, development of clinical judgment and decision-making skill (critical thinking), refinement of skills for clinical practice, and incorporation (by students) of professional nursing values and ethical standards and principles. Thus, knowledge, judgment, skills, values, and ethical reasoning related to the growing population of individuals with development disabilities are essential components, regardless of the level of education (undergraduate, graduate, prelicensure, and advanced practice, among others). Benner and colleagues[46(p29)] have emphasized the importance of integration of knowledge, skill, and "ethical comportment" in nursing education and further emphasize the crucial nature of situated learning—learning in context. From this perspective, presenting information or discussing theories or models of care for individuals with DDs is not adequate; students in the classroom (or in the virtual classroom online) need to be able to place these in context, make meaning of them, and to further explore these meanings through guided practice experiences (eg, clinical experiences and simulations) with faculty who have the necessary expertise and in settings that model best practices in the care of people with DDs. To help students create meaning from facts, evidence, and theories about children and adults with DDs, cases developed by faculty or extrapolated from clinical practice for use in classroom discussions in a wide variety of courses could easily incorporate both nursing care issues and DD concepts. For example, the patient in a case study addressing nursing or APN management of pneumonia in adults could be an individual with autism or Down syndrome. The virtual/computer-driven applications described in the literature (discussed later) are exemplars of similar approaches.

Nursing programs can capitalize on the evolving availability and sophistication of human simulation to provide guided practice experiences to complement clinical practicum encounters with people with DD. Standardized patient simulation cases could offer APN students experiences interacting with and diagnosing actors trained to portray teens or adults with DDs or cognitive disabilities presenting with acute health problems, collaborating with an interdisciplinary developmental team, or interacting with actors portraying families of individuals with DDs. High-fidelity simulation cases could require prelicensure students to care for an adult simulation mannequin designated as having a DD and, in addition, communicate with a family member as portrayed, perhaps, by a faculty member or graduate student, about an individual's care. Clinical decision making and ethical considerations can be integrated in any of these cases or simulation experiences. Exposure to individuals of various ages who have DDs is also important, and students specializing in adult/geriatric care should be well-primed to developed competencies for their care.

Some approaches to the incorporation of DDs content and clinical experience into health professions and nursing curricula have been described in the nursing education literature over the past 10 years. These are summarized below. Research-based evidence of effectiveness of such strategies is limited. More is needed.

DESCRIPTIVE REPORTS OF EDUCATIONAL STRATEGIES

Guillette[47] proposed a curriculum model to promote the development of competencies for home care of children with DDs. Based on a family-centered care and health promotion framework, she recommended formally addressing specific concepts. These included basic skills and knowledge, pathophysiologic bases for pediatric conditions, assessment and communication skills, cultural competence, financing of health care, home care principles, and state and federal law. This model focused primarily, however, on competencies for home care rather than on competencies related to DDs. Hahn's review[3] summarized the development of several computer and Web-based educational projects designed to teach DD concepts to nurses. Ailey and O'Rourke[48,49] designed an undergraduate/graduate nursing student public health experience, based on a community partnership model, for senior prelicensure students and family nurse practitioner (APN) students. Both levels of students had placements at a community agency serving individuals with DDs across the life span. Students, in collaboration with community members, assessed community needs, developed programs, and provided care at the aggregate and individual levels.

Specific objectives and activities varied according to the level of student. Harrison and LaForest[28] described 2 undergraduate nursing clinical placements in which students were directly involved with care of developmentally disabled children. One experience involved the placement of selected students at a residential summer camp for children with special health care needs. In collaboration with their clinical instructor, who functioned as the camp nurse, students provided care for a caseload of children with DDs or other special health care needs. The second clinical experience involved nursing student–kinesthesiology student partnerships for care of a child with a DD enrolled in a sensory-motor stimulation program.

RESEARCH ON EDUCATIONAL STRATEGIES

Sanders and colleagues[43] reported that computer-based instruction using virtual cases improved the knowledge and level of comfort of undergraduate nursing students as related to needs of children with DDs and families. In another article, Sanders and other colleagues[50] reported similar results with nurse practitioner students. Similarly, Boyd and colleagues[51] reported that medical, APN, and physician assistant students had improved knowledge and decreased levels of perceived difficulty of diagnosing and caring for women with intellectual disabilities after completing a computer-based educational program using a virtual case. Tracy and Iacono[45] reported that a training session, which included a brief communication interaction with an individual with a DD, was associated with significantly more positive attitudes toward people with DDs by Australian medical students. Goddard and colleagues[27] reported findings of an action research study in which nursing students were matched by interests, location, and previous experiences with families of children with DDs and worked with them during an 80-hour clinical experience in the United Kingdom. Students partnered with families and parents in particular to support achievement of health goals established by the family. The investigators described 3 major themes as findings from the study: awareness of family health problems, understanding of the family experience of having a child with a DD, and valuing of the family's role and expertise in caregiving.

The few strategies described in the recent literature to support student learning and attitude change related to DDs are weighted somewhat toward the pediatric population, although a few strategies address the interface describe interface between students and adults with DDs. Gaps in understanding of best practices for APN and other graduate students and especially to support development of competencies for interdisciplinary team collaboration are also evident. Little is known about the way that the attitude and knowledge changes reported in the literature will translate to clinical practice (ie, which behaviors and practice patterns will be used by students and graduates of the programs) and, more importantly, whether the outcomes of more comprehensive and better integrated DD content and experiences will improve health outcomes and the health care experience for the population.

SUMMARY

It is challenging to create curricula to prepare nurse graduates of prelicensure and graduate programs to meet the health care needs of a widely diverse constituency whose characteristics and needs are constantly changing. This means that curricula are constantly changing in concert with emerging health considerations and problems. As the population of people with DDs, such as autism, continues to grow, nurses prepared in prelicensure and graduate programs will be increasingly likely to care for them across settings and across the life span. Consider that the prevalence of autism is estimated at 1:88 in 8-year old children and the prevalence of any DD is estimated at 1:6 children, whereas the prevalence of tetralogy of Fallot, a congenital heart defect typically discussed in detail in a prelicensure program, is estimated at 1:2518 live births.[5–7,14] It is increasingly important, and increasingly urgent, for undergraduate and graduate faculty to ensure that competencies for caring for individuals with DDs are addressed adequately in nursing education. Effective educational strategies that target knowledge and attitudes might be supplemented by strategies that promote exposure of students to people of all ages with DDs (ie, planned rather than incidental clinical experiences) and by leveraging evolving and increasingly available human simulation modalities. It is necessary continue to generate evidence about effective ways to help students develop competencies to provide health care services to a growing population of individuals and their families, all of whom often have complex needs and difficulty navigating health care and other resources. The desired outcome of this enterprise is the reduction of health disparities, improved health, and more positive experiences in the health care system for people of all ages with DDs and their families.

REFERENCES

1. Developmental Disabilities and Bill of Rights Act of 2000. 114 STAT. 1684 PUBLIC LAW 106-402-OCT. 30, 2000 section 8. Available at: http://www.acf.hhs.gov/programs/add/ddact/DDA.html. Accessed June 20, 2012.
2. Fisher K, Frazer C, Hasson C, et al. A qualitative study of emergency room nurses perceptions and experiences of caring for individuals with intellectual disabilities in the United States. International Journal of Nursing in Intellectual and Developmental Disabilities 2007;3(1). Available at: http://journal.hsmc.org/ijnidd.
3. Hahn JE. Addressing the need for education: curriculum development for nurses about intellectual and developmental disabilities. Nurs Clin North Am 2003;38:185–204.
4. Souders MC, Paul D, Freeman KG, et al. Caring for children and adolescents with autism who require challenging procedures. Pediatr Nurs 2002;28(6):555–62.
5. Boyle CA, Boulet S, Schieve LA, et al. Trends in the prevalence of developmental disabilities in U.S. children, 1997–2008. Pediatrics 2011;137(6):1034–42.
6. CDC. 2011. Developmental disabilities increasing in the US. Available at: http://www.cdc.gov/Features/dsDev_Disabilities/. Accessed June 20, 2012.
7. Centers for Disease Control. 2011. Data and statistics for the United States. Available at: http://www.cdc.gov/ncbddd/birthdefects/data.html. Accessed June 20, 2012.
8. Gardner MR. Nursing care in early childhood and adolescence. In: Giarelli E, Gardner MR, editors. Nursing of autism spectrum disorder: evidence-based integrated care across the lifespan. New York: Springer Publishing; 2012. p. 77–80.
9. Fisher KM, Peterson J. The nurse's role in managing transitions and future planning for aging adults with autism and their families. In: Giarelli E, Gardner MR, editors. Nursing of autism spectrum disorder: evidence-based integrated care across thelifespan. New York: Springer Publishing; 2012. p. 387–400.
10. Betz CL, Baer MT, Poulson M, et al. Secondary analysis of primary and preventive services accessed and perceived service barriers by children with developmental disabilities and their families. Issues Compr Pediatr Nurs 2004;27:83–106.
11. Kaiser MY, Giarelli E, Pinto-Martin J. Prevalence, etiology and genetics. In: Giarelli E, Gardner MR, editors. Nursing of Autism Spectrum Disorder: Evidence

Based integrated care across the lifespan. New York: Springer Publishing; 2012. p. 25–43.

12. Larson SA, Lakin KC, Anderson L, et al. Prevalence of Mental Retardation and Developmental Disabilities: Estimates From the 1994/1995 National Health Interview Survey Disability Supplements. American Journal on Mental Retardation 2001;106(3):231–52.

13. Kim NH, Hoyak GE, Chow D. Longterm care of the aging population with intellectual and developmental disabilities. Clin Geriatr Med 2011;27(2): 291–300.

14. Centers for Disease Control. Prevalence of autism spectrum disorders—autism and developmental disabilities monitoring network, 14 sites, United States, 2008. MMWR Surveill Summ 2012;61(3):1–19.

15. American Association on Mental Retardation (AAMR), Nursing Division. Intellectual and developmental disabilities nursing: scope and standards of practice. Silver Spring (MD): Nursesbooks.org; 2004.

16. Nehring WM, Roth SP, Natvig D, et al. Intellectual and developmental nursing: scope and standards of practice. Silver Spring (MD): American Nurses Association and Nursing Division of the American Association on Mental Retardation; 2004.

17. Nehring WM. Directions for the future of intellectual and developmental disabilities as a nursing specialty. International Journal of Intellectual and Developmental Disabilities Nursing 2004;1(1). Available at: http://journal.ddna.org/volumes/volume-1-issue-1/.

18. Bureau of Labor Statistics. 2012. Occupational outlook handbook. Available at: http://www.bls.gov/ooh/Healthcare/Registered-nurses.htm#tab-3. Accessed June 15, 2012.

19. Institute of Medicine [IOM]. The future of disability in America. Washington, DC: The National Academies Press; 2007.

20. Smeltzer S, Dolan MA, Robinson-Smith G, et al. Integration of disability-related content in nursing curricula. Nurs Educ Perspect 2005;26(3):210–6.

21. Health Resources and Services Administration [HRSA]. (2012). Maternal child health training program: lend. Available at: http://mchb.hrsa.gov/training/projects.asp?program=9. Accessed June 15, 2012.

22. Melnyk BM, Hawkins-Walsh E, Beauchesne M, et al. Strengthening PNP curricula in mental/behavioral health and evidence-based practice. J Pediatr Health Care 2010;24(2):81–94.

23. Melville C, Cooper SA, Morrison J, et al. The outcomes of an intervention study to reduce the barriers experienced by people with intellectual disabilities accessing primary health care services. J Intellect Disabil Res 2006;50:11–7.

24. Melville C, Finlayson J, Cooper SA, et al. Enhancing primary care health services for adults with intellectual disabilities. J Intellect Disabil Res 2005;49:190–8.

25. Lennox NG, Kerr MP. Primary health care and people with an intellectual disability: the evidence base. J Intellect Disabil Res 1997;41(Pt 5):365–72.

26. Chenoweth L, Pryor J, Jeon Y, et al. Disability-specific preparation programme plays an important role in shaping students specific attitudes towards disablement and patients with disabilities. Learning in Health and Social Care 2004; 3(2):83–91.

27. Goddard L, Mackey S, Davidson P. Functional clinical placements: a driver for change. Nurse Educ Today 2010;30:398–404.

28. Harrison S, LaForest M. Unique children in unique places: innovative pediatric community clinical. J Pediatr Nurs 2011;26:576–9.

29. Honey M, Waterworth S, Baker H, et al. Reflection in the disability education of undergraduate nurses: an effective learning tool. J Nurs Educ 2006;45(11): 445–53.

30. Matziou V, Galanis P, Tsoumakas C, et al. Attitudes of nurse professionals and nursing students towards children with disabilities: do nurses really overcome children's physical and mental handicaps? Int Nurs Rev 2009;56(4):456–60.

31. Hegge M. Ethical issues in the care of individuals with autism spectrum disorder in the family and the community: hearing the voice of the person with autism at the end of life. In: Giarelli E, Gardner MR, editors. Nursing of autism spectrum disorder: evidence-based integrated care across the lifespan. New York: Springer Publishing; 2012. p. 401–23.

32. Kennedy CH, Juarez AP, Becker A, et al. Children with severe developmental disabilities and behavioral disorders have increased special health care needs. Dev Med Child Neurol 2007;49(12):926–30.

33. Liptak GS, Orlando M, Yingling JT, et al. Satisfaction with primary health care received by families of children with developmental disabilities. J Pediatr Health Care 2006;20(4):245–52.

34. Minnes P, Steiner K. Parent views on enhancing the quality of health care for their children with Fragile X syndrome, autism, or down syndrome. Child Care Health Dev 2009;35(2):250–6.

35. Smeltzer SC, Avery C, Haynor P. Interactions of people with disabilities and nursing staff during hospitalization. Am J Nurs 2012;112(4):30–7.

36. Havercamp SM, Scandlin D, Roth M. Health disparities among adults with developmental disabilities, adults with other disabilities and adults not reporting disability in North Carolina. Public Health Rep 2004;119:419–26.

37. Walsh KK, Hammerman S, Josephson F, et al. Caring for people with developmental disabilities: survey of nurses about their education and experience. Ment Retard 2000;38(1):33–41.

38. Werner S. Assessing female students' attitudes in various health and social professions toward working with people with autism: a preliminary study. Journal of interprofessional care 2011;25:131–7.

39. Byrnes M, Gardner MR. Keep calm and carry on: the school nurse and students on the autism spectrum. In: Giarelli E, Gardner MR, editors. Nursing of autism spectrum disorder: evidence based integrated care across the lifespan. New York: Springer Publishing; 2012. p. 171–94.

40. Smeltzer SC, Robinson-Smith G, Dolen MA, et al. Disability-related content in nursing textbooks. Nurs Educ Perspect 2010;31(3):148–55.

41. Aaberg V. Implicit attitudes of nursing faculty toward individuals with disabilities. Retrieved from Proquest Dissertations and Theses. 2010.

42. Giarelli E, Ruttenberg J, Segal A. Continuing education for nurses in the clinical management of autism spectrum disorders: results of a pilot evaluation. J Contin Educ Nurs 2012;43(4):169–76.

43. Sanders CL, Kleinert HL, Free T, et al. Caring for children with intellectual and developmental disabilities: virtual patient instruction improves students' knowledge and comfort level. J Pediatr Nurs 2007;22(6):457–65.

44. Barr JJ, Bracchitta K. Effects of contact with individuals with disabilities. J Psychol 2008;142(3):225–43.

45. Tracy J, Iacono T. People with developmental disabilities teaching medical students: does it make a difference? J Intellect Dev Disabil 2008;33(4):345–8.

46. Benner P, Sutphen M, Leonard V, et al. Educating nurses: a call for radical transformation. San Francisco (CA): Jossey-Bass; 2010.

47. Guillette SE. Preparing student nurses to provide home care for children with disabilities: a strength-based approach. Home Health Care Manag Pract 2002; 15(1):47–58.
48. Ailey SH, O'Rourke ME. Population health clinical experiences at an agency serving individuals with developmental disabilities. Home Health Care Manag Pract 2008;21(1):9–16.
49. American Association on Intellectual and Developmental Disabilities. FAQ on intellectual disability. Available at: http://www.aaidd.org/content_104.cfm. Accessed June 15, 2012.
50. Sanders CL, Kleinert HL, Free T, et al. Developmental disabilities: improving competence in care using virtual patients. J Nurs Educ 2008;47(2):66–73.
51. Boyd SE, Sanders CL, Kleinert HL, et al. Virtual patient training to improve reproductive health care for women with intellectual disabilities. Journal of Midwifery and Women's Health 2008;53(5):453–60.

Genomic Literacy and Competent Practice

Call for Research on Genetics in Nursing Education

Ellen Giarelli, EdD, MA, BSN, BS[a],*, Marian Reiff, PhD, MSc[b]

KEYWORDS

• Genetics • Genomics • Nursing education • Genetic competencies

KEY POINTS

• This article presents an argument that nurse educators should aggressively conduct educational outcomes research on the translation of genetics core competencies at all levels of clinical practice.

• Assuring genetics and genomic literacy among all nurses is a crucial task for contemporary nursing education programs, because translation to practice depends on appropriate education of the nursing at all levels of practice.

• Nurse educators must establish unambiguous evidence that links the nurse's application of genomic information to improved patient outcomes.

INTRODUCTION

There is no controversy regarding the role of genetics in clinical practice, because all diseases involve a genetic component. There is no dispute that nurses must understand basic concepts of genetics and genomics. Genetics and genomics are a necessary component of nursing curricula. A minimum expectation of graduate nurses is that they are literate, such that they have knowledge of genetics and genomics as these topics relate to, and affect, professional nursing practice.

However, some issues are debatable. One issue concerns the process for including genetics and genomics in nursing curricula in baccalaureate, master, and doctoral educational programs. A specific key question that warrants an evidence-based

Disclosure: The authors do not have a relationship with any commercial company that has a direct financial interest in the subject matter or materials discussed in the article.
The study on CMA testing was funded by the National Human Genome Research Institute of the National Institutes of Health (supplement PA-04-126 to Penn CIGHT grant P50 HG004487).
[a] Department of Doctoral Nursing Programs, College of Nursing and Health Professions, Drexel University, 1505 Race Street, Bellet 526, Philadelphia, PA 19102, USA; [b] Division of Translational Medicine and Human Genetics, Center for the Integration of Genetic Health Care Technologies, Perelman School of Medicine, University of Pennsylvania, 3400 Spruce Street, Penn Tower Room 1112, Philadelphia, PA 19104, USA
* Corresponding author.
E-mail address: Eg446@drexel.edu

Nurs Clin N Am 47 (2012) 529–545
http://dx.doi.org/10.1016/j.cnur.2012.07.006
nursing.theclinics.com

answer is: What is the best way to prepare nurses when relevant and essential genomic information is highly fluid and growing exponentially across content areas?

The purpose of this article is to present an argument for research on the practical outcomes of genetics education in professional nursing programs. The authors propose that nurses should aggressively conduct educational outcomes research on the translation of genetics core competencies at all levels of clinical practice. In particular, the authors call for a systematic examination of the factors, including type of preparation in genetics that would influence graduate nurses' applications of concepts to patient care. The authors refer to the new vision for the future of genomics research as articulated by Green and colleagues[1] as support for their observations. First, genomics is central to health promotion and treatment of disease. Second, the public is exposed continually to genetics information and needs to be assured of its accuracy information. Third, health care providers need more systematic training to stay current. Lastly, the best approach to training in genetics is evidence-based.

GENETICS/GENOMICS IS CENTRAL TO HEALTH PROMOTION AND TREATMENT OF DISEASE

Since the publication of the human genome sequence,[2] genomics has been given a fundamental role in biomedical research. Content in genetics is already an essential component of medical and nursing practice and research, and should be included when planning clinical assessments and diagnostics.

A simple accounting of the publications with a genetics/genomics focus from 1990 to 2011 reveals the exponential increase in literature available to professionals and the public. The publications are predominantly evidence-based and examine genetics from bench with animal models to bedside with pharmacogenomics and gene therapy. Between 1990 and 1995, approximately 56,000 articles related to genetics appeared in print professional journals. From 1996 to 2000, in just 5 years, this number jumped to 80,131, representing a 30% increase. Between the years 2005 and 2011, approximately 184,000 articles on genetics were published, and this number is a 70% increase in publications (**Fig. 1**).

Publications on nursing and genetics followed the trend. Between 1990 and 1995, approximately 1550 articles on the topic of genetics and nursing were published in professional journals. The number increased to 2280 between 1996 and 2000. The most significant increase occurred between the years 2005 and 2011. During this period, approximately 5862 publications appeared in the literature addressing some

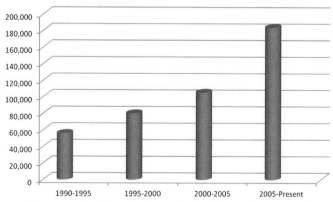

Fig. 1. Frequencies by years of publications in professional journals on topics related to genetics.

topic combining nursing and genetics (**Fig. 2**). Publications with the combined focus of nursing and genomics showed an even greater change over a 21-year period (1990–2011), from 90 to 1663; this is an increase of 1800%. The frequencies illustrate the growing importance of genetics to health care and suggest that nurses are recognizing and realizing their expanded role.

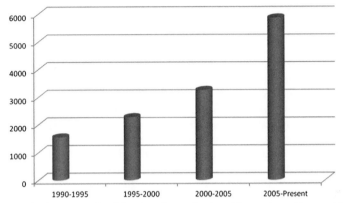

Fig. 2. Frequencies by years of publications in professional journals on the combined topics of nursing/nurses and genetics.

Integration of Genetics into Clinical Care

Genomic information is collected as part of the standard of cancer care.[3,4] Cancer therapies can be identified and prescribed based on the genetic profiles of a patient's tumor or tumor subtype.[5,6] Clinical assessment for conditions such as certain kinds of cancer (eg, HER2 positive) are now and will increasingly in the future incorporate personal genomic information.[7] Rapid genomic analysis of tumors may lead to routine use of genomics-based diagnostics. Drug therapy, guided by genomic information, is quickly becoming the standard of care in anticoagulant therapy.[8] Nurses will likely lead point-of-care implementation of advances in clinical genomics.

Even though considerable evidence from clinical trials is needed before broaching clinical introduction, Green and Guyer noted that "informed and nuanced policies for health care payer coverage could facilitate provisional implementation while definitive data are accrued."[1] The National Human Genome Research Institute (NHGRI) therefore engaged the scientific community and public stakeholders in their initiative to explore future directions and this is in response to the need for increased understanding as opportunities burgeon to understand the nature of genetic contributions to health and illness. Ultimately, nurses will need to think of patient care in terms of assessment of genetic determinants of disease, phenotype, and the role of complex environments.

Assessment of Genetic Contribution to Health and Illness

As recorded in the National Center for Biotechnology Information, more than 2000 genetics tests are available,[9] and more than 330 genome-based applications have been introduced since 2010.[10] Pharmacogenomic testing is routinely conducted before prescribing and administering, and as a part of monitoring, certain medications such as Coumadin.[11]

Chromosomal microarray as an example
Chromosomal microarray (CMA) testing is a genetics technology that is rapidly gaining importance in clinical diagnostics. Current clinical guidelines recommend CMA testing

for patients with clinical phenotypes such as intellectual disability, developmental delay, structural birth defects, and autism.[12,13] CMA allows for improved rate of detection of genomic alterations, and it can be seen as a precursor to genome sequencing.[13] However, many variations are detected that have unknown clinical significance, and with the use of CMA on the rise, there is an increased potential for uncertainty when results are equivocal.[13–15] A clinician with limited understanding of the technology finds it especially difficult to interpret these results and even more difficult to explain to a patient. A recent study examined the perspectives of parents whose children were tested using CMA.[16] Semistructured interviews were conducted with the parents of 25 children who had undergone CMA testing. Qualitative analyses suggested that parents experienced multiple uncertainties with respect to CMA results. They reported that receiving results from health providers lacking genetics expertise contributed to misunderstandings about the meaning of the test results. Results tended to be clarified in consultations with genetics professionals, but several parents reported long waits for genetics consultations, during which time their confusion and anxiety were exacerbated by misinformation gleaned from Internet searches based on inaccurate understandings of the test results. Additionally, parents needed help coping with the implications of genetic results for their child, themselves, and other relatives, and help understanding how the new genetics information could be integrated with their medical care. A professional with proven competency in genetics and genomics will be able to assist patients who experience psychological distress as a consequence of uncertain or disturbing findings. The competent professional will have the knowledge to refer patients to support groups and genetics services.

Therapeutics

Perhaps the single most important role of practicing nurses is their application of genomic therapeutics to patient care. With the increase in pharmaceuticals that rely on genomic information, nurses must understand how to evaluate efficacy, pharmacogenomics, and adverse events given a patient's genomic profile and pharmacodynamics. They must be able to collect accurate data and report behavioral information that plays a role in genotype-specific effects of interventions.[17] This is described as the correlation of genomic signatures with therapeutic response. Observation at the bedside is key.[18]

GENETICS IN POPULAR CULTURE AND PUBLIC DISCOURSE

From early childhood to adult life, the public is exposed continually to genetics through education and popular culture.[19] A broadsheet report of new therapies and advances in genetics may be superficial and confusing to patients. Genetic imagery in the media and popular culture is not necessarily accurate; instead it may be contrived to deliver a message that is political, popular, or provocative. This is illustrated by the spate of image text (cartoons) about cloning and stem cells that appeared in popular literature between 2000 and 2004.[20] As exposure to genetics and genomics increases in a popular forum, the public will likely reach out to nurses for more information and clarification of confusing concepts and explanations of relevance. Nurses are the most prevalent and available health care provider.

Early Education in Genetics

Opportunities to learn about genetics begin in grades Kindergarten through 12. The National Science Education Standards (NSES) proved the basis for State-Of-The-Science standards and indicate which genetics concepts students should learn within the clustered grade levels Kindergarten through 4, 5 through 8, and 9 through 12.[21] In grade levels Kindergarten through 4 and 5 through 8, learning the basic concepts of inheritance and reproduction is expected, while in grades 9 through 12 the molecular basis of heredity and biologic evolution are covered.[21] Students graduating from high school are expected to have a very basic and broad understanding of genetics.

Approximately 10% of 20 million individuals attending associate or bachelor degree programs in the United States are in the life sciences and health fields,[22,23] suggesting that they experience adequate exposure to genetics. The other 90% of graduates may receive some genetics instruction through courses taken as part of general education requirements. Ninety percent of institutions have such requirements organized under broad curricular groups (eg, natural sciences, social sciences, and humanities/fine arts).[24] Within the natural sciences, undergraduate biology courses for nonscience majors are an ideal opportunity for improving genetics education for the general public. However, according to Bowling and colleagues,[25] there has been little evaluation of genetics instruction in these courses.

Lanie and colleagues[26] predicted that the new genetic knowledge and related applications over the next 10 years will have significant implications for all members of society. With this expectation they interviewed adults in the United States about their knowledge of genetics. They discovered a wide range of knowledge of basic concepts, disparate understanding of terminology, and much frustration and hesitancy when asked about genetics. The disconnect between what the public knows and what they may need to know to fully consent to genetics health care has important implications for public health education.

Moreover, there has been little evaluation of genetics instruction in health science curricula including nursing. A pilot assessment of genetics knowledge (genetics literacy) among a cohort of undergraduate nursing students enrolled in an accredited BSN program revealed the sample (N = 191) was 62% literate in genetics. Genetic literacy was measured using an instrument designed by Bowling and colleagues[25] to measure genetic literacy among undergraduates. These findings suggest that literacy remains low even after students received content in secondary school.

SYSTEMATIC TRAINING FOR HEALTH CARE PROVIDERS

Calls for enhanced education of health care providers dates back to the origins of the Human Genome Project.[27] Clinicians must be sufficiently prepared in genomics to understand when it should be applied and to communicate benefits and limitations to patients. According to Feero and Green,[28] the physician community has not been successful in its attempts to aggressively educate clinicians to use genomic information. They attribute this to 4 interrelated issues that also apply to the nursing community. The reasons are: (1) physicians' perception of a lack of immediate relevance to practice, (2) resistance to advances (eg, testing) that are not simple or easily adopted, (3) awaited evidence from large-scale trials, and (4) demands that compete for limited time for more content in an already dense curriculum.[28]

Results from a recent study of preassessment and postassessment of nurse practitioner knowledge of hereditary colorectal cancer evaluate a specific area of nurses' knowledge of genetics, and as a subset of genetics knowledge, it may be a proxy for the larger body of competencies. Edwards and colleagues[29] reported that few nurse practitioners (39%) were comfortable in identifying red flags for a relatively common hereditary cancer syndrome. Furthermore, as knowledge decreased, comfort decreased. Clinicians who do not have comfort with their knowledge base will be less likely to apply it to practice.

A recent study of health provider knowledge of CMA testing offered evidence to support the claim that health professionals require more education to fully integrate this technology into clinical practice. An online survey was completed by a group of 40 physicians[30] (11 pediatricians, 24 pediatric specialists, and 5 medical geneticists) who had ordered CMA testing for their pediatric patients. When asked whether they felt they needed more education about interpreting and explaining test results to families, the physicians in the study had a mean score of 4.03 (standard deviation [SD] 1.69) on a 6-point Likert scale (1 = definitely no; 6 = definitely yes). The mean score of the nongenetics clinicians was significantly higher compared with the medical geneticists (4.32 ± 1.55 vs 2.0 ± 1.22; $P = .006$). The general pediatricians and pediatric specialists reported that most information about CMA testing and interpretation came from informal conversations with colleagues, rather than systematic education. For example, informal discussion with colleagues was listed as a current source of information about CMA by 94.3% of nongenetics clinicians, while professional journals were listed by only 51.4%, and continuing medical education (CME), rounds or seminars were listed by 45.7%. On the other hand, 100% of medical geneticists listed professional journals and CME rounds or seminars as sources of information. Other studies have also reported that nongenetics medical professionals lack the expertise required for adequate care of patients having genetic testing.[30,31] At the same time, however, there is an insufficient number of medical geneticists and genetic counselors to manage the demand for their services.[32,33] It is feasible to consider the possibility that this responsibility might be taken on by nurses. Moreover, without comprehensive understanding of the technology and validity and reliability of interpretation, providers may face ethical issues and questions about liability. Calzone and colleagues[34(p29)] warned that nurses, other health care professionals and their employers will ultimately face significant liability for failing to incorporate genetic/genomic discoveries into practice.

Strategic Plan for Genetics/Genomics in Health Care

According to Khoury and colleagues,[35] underlying any initiative to systematically include genetics in professional education is the assumption that human health can be improved most effectively by first assuring that professionals understand genome biology and that the public has an understanding of normal biology.[35] In February 2011, the National Human Genome Research Institute announced a plan for genomic medicine that is organized by specific domains that cover bench research to bedside care (**Box 1**). The most fundamental premise is that the best way to improve health is to understand normal genome biology as a basis for understanding disease biology. All the domains are relevant to nursing in several ways, but the most basic tenet is

---

Box 1
Domains for charting the course for genomic medicine

Understanding the structure of genomes

Understanding the biology of genomes

Understanding the biology of disease

Advancing the science of medicine

Improving the effectiveness of health care

Data from Green ED, Guyer MS, National Human Genome Research Institute. Charting a course for genomic medicine from base pairs to bedside. Nature 2011;470:204–13.

that phenotypes (physical and behavioral characteristics) are the result of the complex, dynamic interaction of genes, cells, tissues, organs, and the environment.[1]

In the strategic plan of the National Human Genome Research Institute, Green and Guyer[1] assert that realizing the benefits of genomics will require an "educated public who can understand the implications of genomics for their health care and evaluate the relevant public policy issues". Clinical professionals will need to be trained to work within interdisciplinary teams. They advocate for strengthening primary and secondary education and improving the training of science educators. They recommend that programs are needed to reach out to the public to promote "lifelong public understanding and awareness of the role of genomics in human health and other areas." Finally, they advise that all health care providers acquire competency in genomics to provide services appropriate for their scope of practice. This would include better integration into the curricula as well as into "licensing and accrediting processes." Assuring genetics and genomic literacy among all nurses is a crucial task for contemporary nursing education programs, because translation to practice depends on the level of preparation of the nursing workforce at all levels. Clinicians do not need to become geneticists to competently apply genomic advances to practice and competently educate their patients. To accomplish this modest goal, the American Nurses Association in collaboration with specialty nursing organizations described a set of competencies and standards of practice for nurses with regard to genetics and genomics.[36] The competencies were organized by level of professional practice.

BSN Essentials

In 2006, American Nurses Association defined the essential genetics and genomic competencies for all registered nurses. They were created by consensus among representatives from 45 nursing organizations, the Genetic Alliance and the March of Dimes. A second edition added outcome indicators. The competencies are described in a document published by the American Nurses Association, called *Essentials of Genetic and Genomic Nursing: Competencies, Curricula Guidelines, and Outcome measures*, 2nd edition.[37] The document guides nurse educators in the design and implementation of learning experiences that help students and lifelong professional learners to achieve competency in the delivery of genetic and genomic nursing care. Genetic and genomic competencies are accepted as integral to the practice of all registered nurses regardless of academic preparation, role, specialty, or venue. The essential competencies describe 2 domains: (1) professional responsibilities (**Box 2**), and (2) professional practice (**Table 1**). Each has its own set of behavioral objectives and outcome indicators.[37]

MSN Essentials

Nurses prepared at the master's and doctoral levels are expected to translate genetic and genomic advances into the care of all patients and at advanced levels of practice. Nurses with graduate degrees may provide the leadership in caring for clients who have a genetic condition, concern, or a potential genetic component to their health and disease. Advances in genetics and genomics must therefore be a fundamental component of masters nursing curricula to provide graduate students with the knowledge and skills needed for advanced nursing practice, education, and research.

In 2010, a consensus panel began work on master's level competencies that will be published in 2012.[38] The document identifies the nurse with a graduate degree as any nurse prepared at the master's and/or doctoral level practicing in a clinical or nonclinical role. These competencies would apply to anyone functioning at the graduate level in nursing including, but not limited to, advanced practice registered nurses, clinical nurse leaders, nurse educators, nurse administrators, and nurse scientists.

Box 2
Domain: professional responsibilities

- Recognize when one's own attitudes and values related to genetic and genomic science may affect care provided to clients.
- Advocate for clients' access to desired genetic/genomic services or resources including support groups.
- Examine competency of practice on a regular basis, identifying areas of strength, as well as areas in which professional development related to genetics and genomics would be beneficial.
- Incorporate genetic and genomic technologies and information into registered nurse practice.
- Demonstrate in practice the importance of tailoring genetic and genomic information and services to clients based on their culture, religion, knowledge level, literacy, and preferred language.
- Advocate for the rights of all clients for autonomous, informed genetic- and genomic-related decision making and voluntary action.

From American Nurses Association. Essentials of genetic and genomic nursing: competencies, curricula guidelines, and outcome indicators. 2nd edition. Silver Spring (MD): American Nurses Association; 2008. © 2009 American Nurses Association. All rights reserved.

Table 1
Professional practice domain, essential competency, specific competency, and outcome indicators

Competency	Specific Competency—Example	Outcome Indicator—Example
Nursing assessment: Applying/integrating Genetic and genomic Knowledge	Critically analyzes the history and physical assessment findings for genetic, environmental, and genomic influences and risk factors	Demonstrates the ability to incorporate family history as part of the nursing assessment by documenting key genetic and genomic assessment information including a 3-generation family pedigree
Identification	Identifies credible, accurate, appropriate, and current genetic and genomic information, resources, services, and/or technologies specific to given clients	Evaluates the strengths, limitations, and best use of genetics and/or genomic resources for a client or group of clients
Referral activities	Facilitates referrals for specialized genetic and genomic services for clients as needed	Develops an interprofessional plan of care in collaboration with the client that incorporates genetics and genomics
Provision of education, care, and support	Provides clients with interpretation of selective genetic and genomic information or services	Discusses the role of genetic, genomic, environmental, and psychosocial factors in the manifestation of disease

From American Nurses Association. Essentials of genetic and genomic nursing: competencies, curricula guidelines, and outcome indicators. 2nd edition. Silver Spring (MD): American Nurses Association; 2008. © 2009 American Nurses Association. All rights reserved.

According to the authors, the primary purpose of this document is to identify essential genetic and genomic competencies for individuals prepared at the graduate level in nursing. This includes registered nurses with a master's and/or doctorate in another field functioning in a graduate nursing role. The advanced practice registered nurse is the umbrella term appropriate for a licensed registered nurse prepared at the graduate degree level as a clinical nurse specialist, nurse anesthetist, nurse–midwife, or nurse practitioner.[39,40]

The competencies complement and expand on the existing BSN competencies and scope and standards of practice. The document was reviewed by nursing experts from across specialty organizations, and it contains 38 competencies organized under the major categories of: risk assessment and interpretation; genetic education; counseling; testing and results interpretation; clinical management; ethical, legal, and social (ELSI) issues; professional role; leadership; and research.

Current Approaches to Genetic Education in Nursing

The genetic core competencies were used by the American Association of Colleges of Nursing (AACN) to explore a process for facilitating the integration of genomics into nursing curricula. While the AACN recognized the need for essential or basic competencies as well as those appropriate for advanced practice, it did not specify how such competencies should be taught across curricula. In addition to curricular requirements of anatomy and physiology and microbiology, presently the process of genetics education is primarily by integrating genetics content with other content in each nursing course, as appropriate. Most nursing programs in the United States take an integrated approach to genetics education. Nursing programs and schools have the option of adding a stand-alone course in genetics.

Trends in BSN curricula

In 2011, the authors examined the course catalogs of BSN programs in colleges in the United States to determine how genetics was being taught in the curriculum (**Table 2**). The sample comprised 190 BSN programs in 50 states. The authors divided the states into regions and summarized data on whether the curriculum was integrated or included a required course in genetics for undergraduates. Across US states and regions, 27% of BSN programs offered or required a specific course in genetics to

Table 2
Proposed placement of genetics/genomics content across the BSN curriculum

Content Area Related to Genetics	Place in Curriculum
Evolution and population genetics	Course on genetics and health
Genetics, genomics, epigenetics	Course on genetics and health
Environment/genetics and public health	Course on genetics and health, and integrated
Pharmacogenomics	Course on genetics and health, and integrated
Implications of advances for the nursing profession	Course on genetics and health, and integrated
Ethical, legal, social, and cultural issues and implications	Course on genetics and health, and integrated
Screening and diagnosis of diseases	Integrated
Prevention and treatment of disease	Integrated
Implications of genomic advances for patients	Integrated

undergraduate students. The highest rate (32%) was among programs in western states (Alaska, California, Colorado, Hawaii, Idaho, Montana, Nevada, Oregon, Utah, and Wyoming). The lowest rate (13%) was among programs in southwestern states (Arizona, New Mexico, Oklahoma and Texas). For the programs that did not offer a course, the authors did not measure or assess how this was done or how compared across programs (**Box 3**).

Full integration and the addition of a required course in genetics for all students beginning with undergraduates is difficult when curricula and programs are already dense with other content and electives, respectively. At this time, there are no recommended systematic approaches to assessing the comprehensiveness or effectiveness of the integration of genetics content across curricula. However, there are curriculum tools available to nurse educators to assist them in identifying ways to integrate genetics with other core competencies.

Genetic/Genomic Competency Center for Education

Between 2007 and 2011, nurse educators from the National Cancer Institute initiated a multiphase project to establish a Genetic/Genomic Competency Center for Education (called G2C2). The G2C2 is a transdisciplinary repository of genomics education

---

Box 3
Data on process for inclusion of genetics in BSN curricula in programs of nursing in the United States (n = 190)

National

    Percentage with specific genetics course (51/190) 27%

    Percentage with integrated genetics (139/190) 73%

West (Alaska, California, Colorado, Hawaii, Idaho, Montana, Nevada, Oregon, Utah, Washington, Wyoming) (n = 34)

    Percentage with specific genetics course (11/34) 32%

    Percentage with integrated genetics (23/34) 68%

Southwest (Arizona, New Mexico, Oklahoma, Texas) (n = 16)

    Percentage with specific genetics course (2/16) 13%

    Percentage with integrated genetics (14/16) 87%

Midwest (Iowa, Illinois, Indiana, Kansas, Michigan, Minnesota, Missouri, Nebraska, North Dakota, Ohio, South Dakota) (n = 50)

    Percentage with specific genetics course (13/50) 26%

    Percentage with integrated genetics (37/50) 74%

Southeast (Alabama, Arkansas, Florida, Georgia, Kentucky, Louisiana, Mississippi, North Carolina, South Carolina, Tennessee, Virginia, West Virginia) (n = 48)

    Percentage with specific genetics course (15/48) 31%

    Percentage with integrated genetics (33/48) 69%

Northeast (Connecticut, Delaware, Maine, Maryland, Massachusetts, New Hampshire, New Jersey, New York, Pennsylvania, Rhode Island, Vermont) (n = 42)

    Percentage with specific genetics course (10/42) 24%

    Percentage with integrated genetics (32/42) 76%

resources that uses a Web-based management system.[41] This resource has organized materials by discipline (eg, nursing, genetic counseling, physician assistants). It is searchable by competency and performance indicator and links to learning activities and instructional tools. The program is interactive and allows users to add resources that are summarily peer reviewed. From 2008 to 2009, with funding from the National Human Genome Research Institute (NHGRI), the University of Virginia created the Web-based architecture for G2C2. The NHGRI provided funding (2010–2012) for the software to facilitate continued modification, expansion, and development of the G2C2 education repository.[42]

PROPOSED BEST PRACTICE NEEDS EVIDENCE

Members of the clinical research roundtable of the Institute of Medicine (IOM) defined 2 equally important phases of translation of bench science to bedside.[43] The first phase is the "transfer of new understandings of disease mechanisms"[43] learned in the laboratory to the development of new diagnostics, therapy, and prevention. The second phase is the translation of results from clinical studies into everyday clinical practice and health care decision making. It is this second phase that will rely most heavily on another, more recent, IOM recommendation to develop and use the nursing workforce to its full potential.

Significant improvements in the effectiveness of health care are not expected for many years, but realistic achievement can be supported through the systematic education of health care providers and researchers. Nurse educators must establish unambiguous evidence that links the nurse's application of genomic information to improved patient outcomes. Evidence of clinical utility will facilitate the efforts of professional nursing to standardize the process of instruction across levels of preparation, institutions, and classrooms.

Future research must describe: students' genetic literacy on entry and completion of their nursing programs; how nurses are applying the information to practice; and factors that influence best practice, if best practice is defined as the implementation of core competencies with clinical practice.

Recommendations

Khoury and colleagues[35] called for an "expanded multidisciplinary research agenda" to address and fully explore ways bench science can and should be translated to patient care, and in particular the steps of evidence-based recommendations, health care systems and prevention programs, and population health. Central to this intention is the preparation of nurses in the core competencies of responsible practice in the age of genomic health care. To this end, the authors recommend that nurses first critically examine the value and outcome of contemporary education in genetics and application in practice and then unite to envision the future of genetics nursing practice and research.

Genetic Literacy

To improve the learning of genetics, there is a need to first assess students' understanding of genetics concepts and their level of genetics literacy (ie, genetics knowledge as it relates to and affects their lives). Nurse educators must assess baseline knowledge of genetics among faculty members and undergraduate and graduate students. There are surveys available to assess genetics literacy. One tool was developed by Bowling and colleagues at the University of Cincinnati, Ohio.[25] The tool was developed to assess the knowledge of undergraduate students taking introductory

Box 4
Items on the GLAI version 2, 2008

1. What is the relationship among genes, DNA, and chromosomes?

2. Which of the following is a consequence of federal legislation enacted in 2008 entitled Genetic Information Non-Discrimination Act (GINA)?

3. Adult height in people is partially determined by their genes. When environmental conditions are held constant, people have a wide variety of heights (not just short, medium, and tall). Height is probably influenced by:

4. Our understanding of how genes function indicates that:

5. Molecular genetic engineering is possible, because:

6. Which of the following is incorrect regarding meiosis?

7. Sometimes a trait seems to disappear in a family and then reappear in later generations. If neither parent has the trait, but some of the offspring do, what can be concluded about the inheritance of the trait?

8. An individual is found to have a mutation in a gene associated with breast cancer. In which cells is this form of the gene located?

9. Mutations in DNA occur in the genomes of most organisms, including people. What is the most important result of these mutations?

10. Multiple genes are associated with complex diseases such as cancer and mental disorders. When an individual is tested for these genes, what do the results indicate?

11. Which of the following is a current benefit of the application of genetics and genetic technology to health care?

12. A woman has been told she carries a mutation associated with breast cancer. How does this influence her likelihood of developing breast cancer?

13. Many geneticists study the genetic material of organisms such as mice, fruit flies, and yeast. They are able to apply what they learn from these organisms to people, because virtually all different types of organisms are:

14. As human immunodeficiency virus (HIV) has spread around the world, it has become known that some individuals are resistant to the effects of the virus even though they are HIV positive. Why?

15. Which of the following is a characteristic of mutations in DNA?

16. What is the relationship between DNA and chromosomes in higher organisms?

17. Huntington disease is a genetic disorder caused by a dominant gene. Symptoms begin in adulthood, and the disease is ultimately fatal. What is an ethical dilemma presented by Huntington disease when a parent is diagnosed with the disease?

18. Regarding complex traits such as IQ, lung cancer, prostate cancer, and others, how do geneticists describe the contributions of one's genetic makeup and the environment?

19. How is the expression of genes regulated or controlled?

20. If an individual has a genetic test for a mutation causing a particular disease, and the result is positive, what will that most likely mean?

21. What effect, if any, does an individual's environment have on the development of his or her traits?

22. Muscle cells, nerve cells, and skin cells have different functions, because each kind of cell:

23. At what times during an individual's life does the environment influence the expression of his or her genes?

24. Which of the following is incorrect regarding the genetic differences among ethnic groups?

25. What is the relationship between genes and traits expressed in individuals?
26. Which of the following does not accurately reflect Charles Darwin's basic principles of evolution?
27. Which of the following is not considered an ethical or legal concern?
28. Cystic fibrosis (CF) is a recessive disorder, meaning that an individual must have 2 copies of an abnormal CF gene to be affected. What is the probability that a child of 2 individuals who each have one copy of the abnormal gene will be affected with CF?
29. Which of the following is a correct statement about science and the scientific method?
30. The muscle cells of people contain 46 chromosomes. How many chromosomes do unfertilized human egg cells contain?
31. What is an example of an unexpected consequence when current genetic technologies are used?

From Bowling BV, Acra L, Wang L, et al. Development and evaluation of a Genetic Literacy Assessment Instrument for undergraduates. Genetics 2008;178:15–22.

biology or genetics courses, as is the case with BSN students. The Genetic Literacy Assessment Inventory (GLAI) is a 31-item multiple-choice test that addresses 17 concepts identified as central to genetics literacy. The items were selected and modified on the basis of reviews by 25 genetics professionals and educators (**Box 4**). The GLAI is therefore a suitable instrument to assess the need for supplemental education among nursing students who have taken prerequisite biology courses.

It is important to assess student understanding of basic genetics concepts upon entry into nursing programs and on completion of these programs. By doing this we can evaluate the effectiveness of instruction. We can make recommendations for changes to curricula in order to assure that nursing program graduates are at minimum literate with respect to genetics and genomics. The GLAI can be used to evaluate specific knowledge deficits among subgroups of students and within and across course.

Implementation of Core Competencies

At this time, there are no studies that report on how and when graduate nurses apply genetics concepts to their clinical practice. It is not known if and how competencies are consistently performed. Most importantly, it is not known if the application of genetic competencies has an impact on patient outcomes. These conspicuous gaps in information stand between the proposed ideal and the realization of competent nursing practice.

Furthermore, an urgent pedagogical question is: What approach to genetics education produces the desired outcomes of competency and application to practice? Is an integrated curriculum sufficient, or does the addition of a required course make a difference in competencies? Nursing programs will and should continue to include genetics contents. These same programs must be assessed for their impact on nurse behaviors. The value of the pedagogy should be assessed in terms of validity and reliability in affecting best practice nursing care. Nursing education that is designed systematically and based on legitimate evidence of effectiveness will be most flexible. With an evidence-based model of genetics instruction, teachers will be able to respond to rapidly evolving science (genetics) and technology.

An example of a flexible curriculum model is a 2-tiered approach including a required course in genetics and full integration of genetics content across courses. Emphases can be adjusted and adapted to incorporate innovations and advances (**Table 3**). This

Table 3 Two-tiered approach to genetics instruction in BSN curriculum	
Tier in Nursing Curriculum	**Adapted in Response to Changes**
Required course in genetics and health care	Advances in understanding of structure of genomes
	Advances in understanding biology of genomes
	Advances in understanding epigenetics, microbiome
	Genome/health databases
	Advances in metrics for genomic health care
	Advances in population screening and diagnosis
	Evolving approaches to biobanking and patient research
	Public perceptions and direct to consumer marketing of genetic tests (DTC)
Integrated	Advances in improving effectiveness of health care
	Public knowledge and patient education
	Advances in science of genomic medicine and nursing
	Advances in applied pharmacogenomics
	Advances in screening and diagnostics

2-tiered approach can be applied to genetics instruction in BSN curricula. Furthermore, the principle of a 2-tiered approach may also be applied to advanced nursing education.

SUMMARY

Nurses must shift into a gear that is different and proactive.[44] They must fully engage with their peers in the process of incorporating complex genomic information into their teaching. After comparing patients' perceptions of physician and nurse expertise in genetics and clinical outcome, Barnoy and colleagues[45] reported that for the public to accept a nurse's recommendation on genetics testing, the nurse had to be perceived as an expert. Nurses are the main resource to patients who request additional information, and therefore nurses must quickly become experts to positively affect patient outcomes.

As nurses proceed to identify a comprehensive health care agenda that includes nursing research and clinical practice, they will need to examine, through the lens of nursing care, the interactions of genes with other factors that contribute to disease and treatment outcomes. As nurses are the largest cohort of health care providers, they should be poised to deliver intensive environmental or behavioral interventions that are targeted for high-risk groups. If the authors' recommendations are implemented, colleagues in medicine, genetic counseling, and public health could trust that the nursing profession, at large, would have the fundamental educational preparation needed to understand, interpret, and apply advances in genetic technology. With trust and collaboration, together, this would provide the best chance of ensuring that new interventions reach the population for whom they were designed. Genomics will achieve full potential to improve health when "the advances it engenders become accessible to all."[1]

ACKNOWLEDGMENTS

The authors thank Michelle Savard and Mrinalini Sharma for their assistance collecting and analyzing data for this manuscript. The authors are grateful to the Cytogenomics Laboratory and the physicians of Children's Hospital of Philadelphia for granting access to patients and families, and to all the individuals who participated in the research. In addition, the authors appreciate the assistance from Nancy Spinner, Surabhi Mulchandani, Barbara Bernhardt, Reed Pyeritz, Danielle Soucier, and Katherine Ross with the conduct of the research study.

REFERENCES

1. Green ED, Guyer MS, National Human Genome Research Institute. Charting a course for genomic medicine from base pairs to bedside. Nature 2011;470:204–13.
2. International Human Genome Sequencing Consortium. Finishing the euchromatica sequence of the human genome. Nature 2004;431:931–45.
3. Harris L, Fritsche H, Mennel R, et al. American Society of Clinical Oncology 2007 update of recommendations for the use of tumor markers in breast cancer. J Clin Oncol 2007;25:5287–312.
4. Allegra CJ, et al. American Society of Clinical Oncology provisional clinical opinion: testing for KRAS gene mutations in patients with metastatic colorectal carcinoma to predict response to anti-epidermal growth factor receptor monoclonal antibody therapy. J Clin Oncol 2009;27:2091–6.
5. van de Vijver MJ, et al. A gene-expression signature as a predictor of survival in breast cancer. N Engl J Med 2002;347:1999–2009.
6. Paik S, et al. A multigene assay to predict recurrence of tamoxifen-treated, node-negative breast cancer. N Engl J Med 2004;351:2817–26.
7. Ashley EA, Butte AJ, Sheeler MT, et al. Clinical assessment incorporating a personal genome. Lancet 2010;375(9725):1525–35.
8. Rieder MJ, et al. Effect of VKORC1 haplotypes on transcriptional regulation and warfarin dose. N Engl J Med 2005;352:2285–93.
9. National Center for Biotechnology Information. GeneTests. Available at: http://www.ncbi.nlm.nih.gov/sites/GeneTests?db=GeneTests. Accessed January 15, 2012.
10. Gwinn M, Grossnicklaus DA, Yu W, et al. Horizon scanning for new genomic tests. Genet Med 2011;13(2):161–5.
11. Frueh FW, et al. Pharmacogenomic biomarker information in drug labels approved by the United States Food and Drug Administration: prevalence of related drug use. Pharmacotherapy 2008;28:992–8.
12. Manning M, Hudgins L. Array-based technology and recommendations for utilization in medical genetics practice for detection of chromosomal abnormalities. Genet Med 2010;12(11):742–5.
13. Miller DT, Adam MP, Aradhya S, et al. Consensus statement: chromosomal microarray is a first-tier clinical diagnostic test for individuals with developmental disabilities or congenital anomalies. Am J Hum Genet 2010;86(5):749–64.
14. Kohane IS, Masys DR, Altman RB. The incidentalome: a threat to genomic medicine. JAMA 2006;296(2):212–5.
15. Redon R, Ishikawa S, Fitch KR, et al. Global variation in copy number in the human genome. Nature 2006;444(7118):444–54.
16. Reiff M, Bernhardt BA, Mulchandani S, et al. "What does it mean?": uncertainties in understanding results of chromosomal microarray testing. Genet Med 2012;14:250–8.
17. McBride CM, et al. Future health applications of genomics: priorities for communication, behavioral, and social sciences research. Am J Prev Med 2010;38:556–65.
18. Caskey CT. Using genetic diagnosis to determine individual therapeutic utility. Annu Rev Med 2010;61:1–15.

19. Lindee S, Nelkin D. The DNA mystique: the Gene as a cultural icon. Ann Arbor (MI): University of Michigan Press; 2004.
20. Giarelli E. Images of cloning and stem cell research in editorial cartoons. Qual Health Res 2006;16:61–78.
21. National Research Council. National science education standards. Washington, DC: National Academy Press; 1996.
22. National Center for Education Statistics. Total fall enrollment in degree-granting institutions, by control and type of institution, age, and attendance status of student: 2009. Digest of educational statistics, 2010. Available at: http://nces.ed.gov/programs/digest/d10/tables/dt10_201.asp?referrer=list. 2010. Accessed August 9, 2012.
23. National Center for Education Statistics. Degrees in the health professions and related sciences conferred by degree- granting institutions, by level of degree and sex of student: 1970-71 through 2008-09. Available at: http://nces.ed.gov/programs/digest/d10/tables/dt10_322.asp?referrer=list. Accessed August 9, 2012.
24. Hurtado S, Astin AW, Dey EL. Varieties of general education programs: an empirically based taxonomy. J Gen Educ 1991;40:133–62.
25. Bowling BV, Acra L, Wang L, et al. Development and evaluation of a Genetic Literacy Assessment Instrument for undergraduates. Genetics 2008;178:15–22.
26. Lanie AD, Jayaratne TE, Sheldon JP, et al. Exploring the public understanding of basic genetic concepts. J Genet Couns 2004;13(4):306–19.
27. Collins FS. Preparing health professionals for the genetic revolution. JAMA 1997; 278(15):1285–6.
28. Feero WG, Green ED. Genomics education for health care professionals in the 21st century. JAMA 2011;306(9):989–90.
29. Edwards QT, Maradiegue A, Seibert D, et al. Pre-/postassessment of nurse practitioner's knowledge of hereditary colorectal cancer. J Am Acad Nurse Pract 2011;23:361–9.
30. Kegley J. An ethical imperative: genetics education for physicians and patients. Med Law 2003;22(2):275.
31. Harvey EK, Fogel CE, Peyrot M, et al. Providers' knowledge of genetics: a survey of 5915 individuals and families with genetic conditions. Genet Med 2007;9(5):259–67.
32. Greendale K, Pyeritz RE. Empowering primary care health professionals in medical genetics: how soon? How fast? How far? Am J Med Genet 2001; 106(3):223–32.
33. Grody WW. Ethical issues raised by genetic testing with oligonucleotide microarrays. Mol Biotechnol 2003;23(2):127–38.
34. Calzone K, Cashion A, Feetham SL, et al. Nurses transforming health care using genetics and genomics. Nurs Outlook 2010;58(1):26–35.
35. Khoury MJ, Gwinn M, Bowen S, et al. Beyond base pairs to bedside: a population perspective on how genomics can improve health. Am J Public Health 2012; 102(1):34–7.
36. Daack-Hirsch S, Dieter C, Quinn Griffin MT. Integrating genomics into undergraduate nursing education. J Nurs Scholarsh 2011;43(3):223–30.
37. American Nurses Association. Essentials of genetic and genomic nursing: competencies, curricula guidelines, and outcome indicators. 2nd edition. Silver Spring (MD): American Nurses Association; 2008.
38. Greco KE, Tinley S, Seibert D. Essential genetic and genomic competencies for nurses with graduate degrees- draft document. Silver Springs (MD): American Nurses Association and International Society of Nurses in Genetics; 2012.

39. National Council of State Boards of Nursing. The consensus model for APRN regulation: licensure, accreditation, certification, and education. Available at: https://www.ncsbn.org/aprn.htm. Accessed August 9, 2012.

40. Greco KE, Tinley S, Seibert D. Essential genetic and genomic competencies for nurses with graduate degrees— draft document. Silver Springs (MD): American Nurses Association; 2011.

41. Calzone K, Jerome-D'Emilia B, Jenkins J, et al. Establishment of the Genetic/ Genomic Competency Center for Education. J Nurs Scholarsh 2011;43(4):351–8.

42. Genetic/Genomic Competency Center for Education (G2C2). Available at: http:// www.g-2-c-2.org/. Accessed August 9, 2012.

43. Sung NS, Crowley WFJ, Genel M, et al. Central challenges facing the national clinical research enterprise. JAMA 2003;289(10):1278–87.

44. Jenkins J, Bednash G, Malone B. Guest editorial: bridging the gap between genomic discoveries and clinical care: nurse faculty are key. J Nurs Scholarsh 2011;43(1):1–2.

45. Barnoy S, Levy O, Bar-Tal Y. Nurse or physician: whose recommendations influence the decision to take genetics tests more? J Adv Nurs 2009;66(4):806–13.

The Doctor of Nursing Practice Graduate as Faculty Member

Sandra Bellini, DNP, APRN, NNP-BC, CNE*,
Paula McCauley, DNP, APRN, ACNP-BC, CNE,
Regina M. Cusson, PhD, NNP-BC, APRN

KEYWORDS

- DNP • Clinical scholarship • Faculty roles

KEY POINTS

- This article focuses on the emerging role of the doctor of nursing practice (DNP) graduate as faculty member.
- Re-evaluation of Boyer's model of scholarship in relation to faculty roles is examined.
- Discussion includes barriers facing current DNP faculty as well as the potential advantages that DNP graduates may make toward school of nursing faculties.

HISTORICAL COMPOSITION OF FACULTY AND TRADITIONAL FACULTY ROLES

Nursing has overcome its roots as an apprentice-based educational system. In the days before Florence Nightingale professionalized nursing, a good nurse was one who showed up clean, sober, and ready to engage in heavy manual labor. Miss Nightingale created an education system for training nurses in 1860, with the first secular school of nursing at St. Thomas' Hospital, London, now part of King's College. Miss Nightingale's nurses went on to develop other nursing training programs throughout the world, with training based on an apprenticeship model emphasizing direct care provision as well as teaching.[1]

By the beginning of the twentieth century, preparation as a nurse educator had progressed into the university system, but there were no nursing doctoral programs until the 1970s.[2] Doctoral preparation for nursing faculty was often completed in schools of education, with the first doctoral program awarding an EdD to nurses at Teachers College, Columbia University in 1924.[3] Other nurses pursued doctoral degrees in related fields, such as human development, anthropology, physiology, and other sciences. The first PhD in nursing was awarded by New York University in the 1930s.

Disclosures: None of the authors has a relationship with a commercial company that has a direct financial interest in the subject matter or materials discussed in the article.
School of Nursing, University of Connecticut, 231 Glenbrook Road, U-2026, Storrs, CT 06269-2026, USA
* Corresponding author.
E-mail address: sandra.bellini@uconn.edu

Nurs Clin N Am 47 (2012) 547–556
http://dx.doi.org/10.1016/j.cnur.2012.07.004   nursing.theclinics.com
0029-6465/12/$ – see front matter © 2012 Elsevier Inc. All rights reserved.

The 1960s were a time of many milestones for advanced education in nursing. Federal funding was available to nursing doctoral students for the first time, with an emphasis on preparing nurses as scholars and researchers.[4] Nursing specialization developed, setting the stage for nurses to earn doctoral degrees specifically geared to preparation as academicians in a nursing specialty.[2] By the mid-1970s, there was sufficient nursing science developed to support different types of nursing doctoral degrees: the PhD focused on nursing science and the doctor of nursing science (DNS or DNSc) was intended to be more clinically focused. Academic politics played a role in this separation and the preparation at the DNS level was often identical to PhD preparation at other institutions.[3] In recent years, universities have recognized the nature of the original education and converted graduates' degrees to PhDs.

At approximately the same time, preparation as a nurse educator was replaced by increased content in research and nursing science. Where students had previously developed expertise in teaching strategies, often at the master's degree level, the focus shifted to developing content and research expertise. As the PhD replaced the master's degree as the required education for nurse academics, preparation as a teacher disappeared from the curriculum. How PhD-prepared nurses were supposed to learn how to teach was not addressed, leaving many new faculty members unprepared to develop their courses and teach their classes. Universities began offering on-the-job training to prepare their new scholars to succeed in the classroom; however, a pedagogical base and knowledge was often lacking in curriculum development. Recent trends include a return to education courses as electives in the doctoral curriculum.

Nurses still sought an opportunity to earn a doctoral degree that would focus on clinical expertise and scholarship. Many expert nurses did not want to leave clinical nursing for the realms of the classroom and of knowledge generation and theory development. The DNP has begun to fill that void. The origin and merits of the DNP degree have been discussed extensively elsewhere. One decision, however, that became part of The Essentials of Doctoral Education for Advanced Nursing Practice[5] had a major impact on the content of DNP education. Teaching expertise was left out of that document. DNP graduates were not prepared to be educators, in spite of a shortage of nursing faculty. A window remained slightly open, however, by indicating that DNPs could seek preparation as educators outside of their doctoral program. The Research Council of The National Academies, in their 2005 report, Advancing the Nation's Health Needs: NIH Research Training Programs, indicated that a clinical doctorate in nursing similar to the MD and PharmD degrees could ameliorate the shortage of clinical faculty.[6] As DNP-prepared graduates enter the workplace, schools of nursing are common employers. The number of graduates with DNP degrees exceeded the number with PhD degrees for the first time in 2011.[7] Who better to teach the DNPs of tomorrow than DNP-prepared educators?

THE ARRIVAL OF THE PRACTICE SCHOLAR IN THE ACADEMIC SETTING

DNP-prepared educators make the link between education and practice. DNP-prepared faculty want to remain in clinical practice: that was often the reason that they sought a DNP degree. As the demands of research output increased for PhD-prepared faculty, they most often left the clinical practice arena. Clinical knowledge changes rapidly over time, so nurse academics are often disconnected from the clinical world. Choices must be made in the pursuit of academic progression, and active clinical practice is often discarded. This creates a disconnect between what is taught in the classroom and what is happening in clinical practice. DNP-prepared nurse educators can change that scenario. As clinically active nurse educators,

DNP-prepared nurse educators can infuse cutting-edge practice knowledge into the nursing curriculum and make a major contribution to bridging the education–practice gap. It must also be remembered that DNP-prepared nurse educators are prepared as clinical scholars, who will disseminate practice-based scholarship. The potential for relevancy of nursing scholarship is enhanced with the incorporation of DNP-prepared clinical scholars into the academic setting.

Research partnerships between PhD-prepared and DNP-prepared faculty are a logical outcome of employing both types of graduates in schools of nursing. PhD-prepared educators bring research expertise and DNP-prepared educators bring practice expertise. Both areas of expertise are greatly needed to solve societal health problems. By working together, blending areas of knowledge and expertise, educators can reach their greatest potential.

BOYER'S MODEL OF SCHOLARSHIP REVISITED

Dialogue and attempts to define what does and does not constitute "scholarship" in academic settings is not a new phenomenon. Since 1990, with the publication of Boyer's model, based on his study funded by the Carnegie Foundation for the Advancement of Teaching,[8] the various forms of scholarship as described by Boyer have been discussed, dissected, debated, and subsequently endorsed by many colleges and universities across the United States. According to Boyer, the 4 types of scholarship are defined as discovery, integration, application, and teaching.

The first type of scholarship, discovery, is consistent with the gold standard of traditional research within an academic community. Discovery research focuses on the generation of knowledge for its own sake, therein worthy of intellectual pursuit. As an example, the contributions of traditional nursing faculty, through discovery research, have provided the foundation for the establishment of nursing as a respected discipline within the academic setting and, with that, the recognition that nursing faculty are scholars in their own right.

The scholarship of integration can be described as the ability to connect concepts and therefore give meaning to various facts or the ability to interpret what groups of various findings mean when put into context. An example of this is the role of the nurse practitioner, who assesses patient history; conducts comprehensive physical examinations; orders laboratory work, appropriate radiology studies, and so forth; and integrates those findings to develop differential diagnoses and subsequent plan of care for patients. Through her actions, she integrates findings from the disciplines of medicine, nursing, pharmacy, and other behavioral and social sciences.

The scholarship of application, as put forth by Boyer, raises the notion that the first 2 forms of scholarship should contribute their collective knowledge toward the greater good of society.[8] The idea is that knowledge, once discovered, carries with it the social responsibility to share that theoretic knowledge beyond the academic setting where it can then interact with practice in a dynamic way. The result of this translation of theory into practice can, on its own, result in new knowledge. An important distinction to make is that Boyer specifically speaks to what scholarship of application is and is not: it is the intersection and interaction of theory and practice and is not the simple act of taking discovered knowledge and applying it.[8(p3)] A second distinction (discussed later) is that scholarship of application needs to be defined and separated from service; one does not necessarily infer the other.

Service refers to acts of good citizenship, which although important and valuable to a community, may or may not directly relate to scholarship. Conversely, true scholarship of application requires that "service activities must be tied directly to one's special field of knowledge and relate to, and flow directly out of, this professional activity."[8(p22)] Boyer also discusses, in this section of his work, that "all too frequently, service means not doing scholarship but doing good."[8(p22)] This widespread misapplication of the term, *scholarship of application*, may be at the root of problems currently encountered by practicing DNP faculty (discussed later).

The fourth form of scholarship, as described by Boyer, is the scholarship of teaching.[8] The quintessential scholar in this realm is the gifted professor, the educator who is able to convey expert knowledge to students. According to Boyer, scholarship of "teaching both educates and entices future scholars."[8(p23)] In nursing education circles, excellence in teaching is an expectation of all faculty members, research or clinical. In regard to DNP-prepared faculty in particular, the National League for Nursing[9] advocates educational pedagogy in addition to DNP education, a position echoed by the American Association of Colleges of Nursing (AACN).[5,10] In the interest of promoting faculty scholarship, it is difficult to argue with this collective stance.

Of all the disciplines represented on college and university campuses across the nation, nursing, to a large extent, has endorsed Boyer's model.[11–13] In their 1999 publication defining scholarship in nursing, the AACN[12] describes Boyer's model in detail and, more recently, in their publications pertaining to the DNP in particular.[5,10] In light of this background, it is unclear why some faculties are having difficulty with the reconciliation of the concepts of scholarship and clinical practice. It seems that through the AACN references to Boyer's work in the DNP essentials document,[5] that scholarship is an expected outcome of DNP programs, not simply a professional degree conferred without scholarly merit.

BARRIERS FACING DNP FACULTY
Operationalizing the Concept of Clinical Scholarship

Among several significant barriers facing DNP-prepared faculty members, one of the most troublesome is the widespread lack of appreciation and acceptance of clinical scholarship as a worthy endeavor by many traditional nursing faculties. Given that the emphasis in DNP education and role expectation is focused on practice, this is an essential paradigm shift for nursing to make if the collective goal is to further the influence of the discipline. To accomplish this goal requires careful and thoughtful evaluation and redesign of many traditional frames of reference pertaining to exactly what does and does not qualify as nursing scholarship. Perhaps, again, Boyer's model can lend assistance.

Although Boyer used the term, *scholarship of application*, in his 1990 publication, the concepts that inspire the idea have been identified by several other titles over time, including *scholarship of practice*,[14] *clinical scholarship*,[15–17] or, later in life, again from Boyer,[18] who relabeled the concept, *scholarship of engagement*. Whatever the title, several themes are consistent, relevant, and applicable for nursing.

The first recurring theme concerns the word, *practice*. Florence Nightingale's[19] description of the importance of observation in nursing practice laid the groundwork for the qualities later recognized as the hallmark of the expert, reflective nurse or the original clinical scholar. In nursing, the idealized knowledgeable, reflective practitioner is synonymous with Benner's early work in which, she describes the uncovering of knowledge imbedded in the clinical practice of the expert practitioner.[20] As described by Mundinger,[15] a clinical scholar is a "doer," someone actively engaged in practice.

The second recurring theme is the word, *scholarship*. Clinical scholarship, in particular, has emerged as a closely related concept, with many similar definitions.[15–17,21]

Regardless of the particular source cited, clinical scholarship as a concept requires astute observation on behalf of an expert clinician, which provides context, substantial nursing experience, extensive scientific knowledge, and intellectual activity and which can take various forms.[15–17,21,22]

Perhaps what needs to be reconciled is the concept of clinical scholarship with scholarship of application. Although each has its own definitions and qualities, it could be argued that the role of the clinical scholar is to exemplify the qualities consistent with clinical scholarship, thereby embodying the scholarship of application through practice. As Mundinger[15] suggests, clinical scholars are experts actively engaged at the highest levels of practice, the core of the discipline. The practice setting, where the clinical scholar meets patients in a real-world context, is the juxtaposition where theory and practice meet; it is precisely where new knowledge can be generated as described by Boyer,[8] through the application of theory in clinical practice. It is where DNP-prepared faculty can exemplify the role of clinical scholar engaged in scholarship of application through advanced clinical practice.

Role Expectations for DNP Faculty

As more DNP-prepared faculty arrive in the academic setting, several issues need to be considered; among them are appropriate teaching loads. In academic settings where clinical faculty members are not eligible for tenure, teaching loads are often higher than for new faculty hired into a tenure track. Perhaps an alternative and yet mutually satisfactory arrangement to this traditional structure would be to establish different, yet clear and undeniably rigorous, scholarship expectations for DNP-prepared clinical faculty. Assigning new hires a lighter initial teaching loads allows both for time in practice as a joint appointment as well as time for establishment and development of application scholarship. Expected activities for DNP faculty could consist of collaborative educational or clinical research studies, publications, policy work, and advanced practice nursing at the doctoral level (ie, consultation, leadership roles in practice settings, quality improvement, or outcomes management projects). As joint appointees, DNP faculty as envisioned by AACN[5,10] could bring financial support for their salaries to the university setting in much the same way that tenure track faculty bring financial support through research grants. For academic settings not to consider alternative arrangements for DNP faculty is a missed opportunity for nursing to elevate practice-related scholarship within the academic community, which is essential for a practice discipline.

Relationship of DNP Faculty to Clinical Practice: At Your "Service"?

When discussing scholarship of application, an important goal is to build constituencies external to the academic setting.[18] As articulated by the AACN,[5,10] one of the assumed responsibilities for DNP faculty is to remain active in clinical practice and promote the advancement of clinical practices, consistent with the role of the clinical scholar.[15] Within this context, a troubling conundrum exists across many colleges and universities related to scholarship versus service (discussed previously). As Boyer[8] mentions specifically, service does not necessarily require scholarship. Why then should clinical practice at the advanced level, therefore requiring specific knowledge for application, be considered faculty activity equivalent to, for instance, serving on a university planning committee? Although committee work is a worthwhile endeavor, it can hardly be argued that engaging in such committee work is an activity that "must be tied directly to one's special field of knowledge and relate to, and flow directly out of, this professional activity."[8(p22)] Advanced nursing practice is most assuredly tied directly to, relates to, and flows directly out of a specialized field of knowledge, specifically nursing practice knowledge, and is consistent with Boyer's criteria for scholarship. Advanced nursing practice is not an act of charity, nor is it a hobby and should not be equated as such. This foundational assumption, common in many academic settings, will likely remain a challenge for DNP faculty for years to come.

The pursuit of excellence in clinical scholarship is an intellectual activity that should be advocated at the core of professional nursing identity values as a practice discipline. These ideas are not new to nursing; similar sentiments have appeared in the literature in esteemed publications from the AACN,[12] the National Organization of Nurse Practitioner Faculties,[23,24] and Sigma Theta Tau International[21] for more than a decade. If the national organizations seem to share these assertions, it is difficult to understand the lack of progress on this initiative nationally.

With the 2004 position statement on the DNP, the educational pathway that historically has had advanced practice registered nurse (APRN) education at the master of science level seems poised for change.[25] As entry into practice for advanced practice clinicians becomes the DNP, it follows that the educational credentials for advanced practice clinical faculty will also move to the DNP. This is decidedly different from past pathways to advanced practice. The potentially important distinction going forward is that contrary to the past, APRN faculty will be educated as DNPs, not as master of science–level nurse practitioners, who then pursue PhDs as their terminal degree. Over time, today's APRN/PhD-prepared faculty will no longer be the norm, as PhD education becomes largely BS-PhD without encompassing advanced practice content. Clinical programs of the future may ideally be led by clinical scholars active in and committed to practice. Therefore, elevating the level of scholarship expected for clinical faculty to be more consistent with their PhD counterparts makes sense. It is in the professions' best interest to have consistent levels of excellence across doctoral-level education programs and comparable levels of expected scholarship for faculty.

Promotion and Tenure Issues

Although the impetus of Boyer's[8] study was to examine undergraduate education, the use of faculty time in terms of what counted toward tenure and promotion emerged as a significant problem from the faculty perspective. In simple terms, Boyer[8] articulates the need for recognition of 4 types of scholarship and advocates that promotion and tenure decisions be inclusive of the many forms, not exclusively based on the conduct of research, as has been a common practice, especially at universities granting doctoral degrees.[8] Again, these sentiments are echoed in publications that have appeared in the nursing literature for many years.[10,12,21,23,24] Yet, tenure criteria in many research extensive settings still do not reflect this broader description of scholarly activity. As we face faculty shortages and pressures from outside the discipline, is it not time to reconcile professional nursing's identity and embrace both the art and the science that are inherent in nursing?

As long as criteria for tenure are designed to reflect discovery scholarship primarily or exclusively, faculty engaged in scholarship of application will have difficulty with eligibility. These concerns are already appearing in the literature on behalf of current DNP students with future aspirations in education.[26] The challenge for current faculty to accept is that few, if any, DNP faculty coming to the academic setting would advocate eligibility for promotion or tenure without strict, rigorous criteria, rather that the criteria be more reflective of the type of scholarship in which they are to engage. To advocate tenure eligibility for clinical faculty takes nothing away from the wonderful discovery work of traditional research faculty; rather, it expands the visibility of the varied forms that nursing scholarship can take, a position endorsed by AACN.[10] For an applied science discipline firmly rooted in practice, to have to engage in this debate in 2012 remains an ongoing frustration for many of the earliest DNP-prepared APRN faculty to arrive in academic settings.

ADVANTAGES TO SCHOOLS OF NURSING EMPLOYING DNP GRADUATES AS FACULTY

Incorporation of DNPs into faculty at schools of nursing brings numerous advantages. The DNP role encompasses objectives identified in the *Future of Nursing*'s[27] message to ensure that nurses practice to the full extent of their education and training, improve nursing education, provide opportunities for nurses to assume leadership positions and serve as full partners in health care redesign, and improve efforts and improve data collection for workforce planning and policy making. The health care system is in a state of evolution, requiring a dynamic knowledge base of nursing and health science as well as skills in management, education, and organizational systems.[3] The practice doctorate addresses the need for safe practice, the increasing complexity of health care, the need for parity with other disciplines, the continuing explosion of knowledge, and the need for more nursing faculty.[28]

The DNP preparation focus is on practice, which is important to remember in this discussion because nursing is a practice discipline. DNP-prepared nurse faculties focus on the scholarship of integration, application, and teaching of knowledge. The scholarship of DNP graduates is practice-focused in nature, allowing the focus to remain on the evidence base, strengthening evidence-based practice. Benner and colleagues[29] evaluated the current nursing education system and confirmed that there is a need to change the preparation of future nurses. The DNP not only advances the profession but also provides the profession the opportunity to close the gap between education and practice.[30]

The explosion of knowledge in health care provides further evidence of the need for the DNP faculty. The knowledge required to provide leadership in the discipline of nursing is complex and rapidly changing.[3] The education of DNPs includes focus on evaluation and application of research rather than primarily on the conduct of research. DNP education emphasizes scholarly practice, practice improvement, innovation, and testing of interventions and care delivery models, leadership in establishing clinical excellence as well as evaluation of health care outcomes, and expertise to inform heath care policy.[31] By emphasizing a systems perspective, the DNP education equips nurses with the knowledge and skills to solve system issues in their own area of practice. DNP faculty members come prepared with evidence-based arguments and policy skills, having an impact on the many facets of the current health care arena and forthcoming health care reform.

Many DNP faculty members are engaged in practice as an integral part of their role. Faculty practice supports the mission and vision of schools of nursing. Faculty practice sustains practice skills, expands clinical placement sites, and increases quality of clinical education through role models and mentoring. Practice scholars on a nursing faculty provide a value-added component to preparation of the next generation of practitioners.[30] DNP clinical faculty, as active preceptors and health care professionals in their community, reflect the perspective of the community practitioner.[32] DNP-prepared faculty will provide the need for comprehensive preparation of advance practice students. Dissertation requirements or capstone projects grounded in clinical practice and designed to solve practice problems or to inform practice directly create an emphasis on practice. DNP faculties are experts in practice and facilitate these scholarly endeavors.

The DNP provides additional options to nurses seeking a terminal practice-focused degree necessary to educate future nurses. There are differences in the personality characteristics of practitioners and researchers.[33] Clinicians (DNPs) demonstrate integrative thinking patterns, whereas researchers (PhDs) may be reductionists. Clinicians are poised to translate the knowledge into practice that has been generated by the research. DNP scholarship focus is on integration and application of knowledge and is more local and practical.[33] There are similarities and differences in doctorally prepared nurses. Both patterns of thinking are highly valued in nursing and necessary for future nurses to master to close the theory-to-practice gap.[34] DNP-prepared nurses are practitioner–researchers with advanced understanding of health care delivery systems necessary to translate newly discovered knowledge into health care. These characteristics are necessary in faculty toolboxes for comprehensive nursing education.

THE FUTURE OF FACULTY COMPOSITION: LEARNING TO MAKE THE MOST OF COLLECTIVE TALENTS

There is concern for decreased interest in the research degree (PhD) in favor of the DNP, even though the 2 are complementary and overlap.[35] The research mission is to generate knowledge, and the practice mission is to apply that knowledge in clinical practice, as a means of generating new knowledge resulting from the interface of research and practice. The interaction between the 2 supports both degrees. DNP faculty members can be initiators of an idea as well as providers of care and practice partners in research with PhD faculty members. Research questions often are generated through clinical practice, and those questions become the focus of research programs. Researchers can only benefit from the assistance of DNP-prepared faculty in performing the education and service missions of the school. The practice expertise of DNP faculty complement and supplement the research and scholarship of the PhD-prepared faculty.[33] Teams of PhD and DNP nurses have the potential to ask provocative clinical questions and conduct highly relevant research. DNP faculty bring contemporary knowledge of practice issues and access to practice sites incorporating scholarship through translational research. DNP faculty are prepared with greater emphasis on the translation of research into practice supporting the theory–research–application cycle.[30]

SUMMARY

DNP graduates who seek careers in the academic setting do so because they wish to pursue scholarship. The question is, Does the traditional form of scholarship need to remain as strictly prescribed, or is it time to broaden perspectives? Other important questions also remain to be answered: Who are DNP-prepared faculty? How are they philosophically similar and dissimilar to traditional faculty? Are DNP-prepared clinical faculty different from traditional clinical faculty? What expertise can they bring to the academic world? And, probably most importantly, how will nontraditional DNP-prepared faculty assimilate into a world largely designed for more traditional scholars?

Perhaps academicians need to reconceptualize what it means to be a scholar in nursing. Perhaps also, the academic setting needs to reacquaint itself with the roots of the discipline and embrace clinical practice as a worthy intellectual pursuit. Clinical practice, within the context of a practice discipline, should be considered the core of the profession. Clinical practice, reconsidered as the manifestation of scholarship of application and executed by DNP-prepared faculty, is a scholarly endeavor. Perhaps in time, as faculty mixes become more integrated and PhD-prepared and DNP-prepared scholars learn to work collaboratively toward the advancement of the discipline, the 2 descriptors of nursing—art and science—will work more synergisti-cally than in the past.

REFERENCES

1. Bostridge M. Florence nightingale: the woman and her legend. London: Penguin Viking; 2008.
2. Bartels JE. Preparing nursing faculty for baccalaureate-level and graduate-level nursing programs: role preparation for the academy. J Nurs Educ 2007;46(4): 154–8.
3. Apold S. The doctor of nursing practice: looking back, moving forward. J Nurse Pract 2008;4(2):101–7.
4. Marriner-Torney A. Historical development of doctoral programs from the middle ages to nursing education today. Nurs Health Care 1990;11(3):132–7.
5. American Association of Colleges of Nursing. The essentials of doctoral educa-tion for advanced nursing practice. Washington, DC: Author; 2006. Available at: http://www.aacn.nche.edu/DNP/pdf/Essentials.pdf. Accessed April 4, 2012.
6. National Research Council. Advancing the nation's health care needs: NIH research training programs. Washington (DC): National Academies Press; 2005.
7. American Association of Colleges of Nursing. AACN 2011 survey. 2012. Available at: http://www.aacn.nche.edu/news/articles/2012/enrollment-data. Accessed April 4, 2012.
8. Boyer EL. Scholarship reconsidered: priorities of the professoriate. Princeton (NJ): Carnegie Foundation for the Advancement of Teaching; 1990.
9. National League for Nursing. Reflection and dialogue: doctor of nursing practice. 2007. Available at: http://www.nln.org/aboutnln/reflection_dialogue/refl_dial_1.htm. Accessed May 4, 2010.
10. American Association of Colleges of Nursing. The DNP roadmap task force report. Washington, DC: Author; 2006.
11. Starck P. Boyer's multidimensional nature of scholarship: a new framework for schools of nursing. J Prof Nurs 1996;12:268–76.
12. American Association of Colleges of Nursing. AACN position statement on defining scholarship for the discipline of nursing. Washington, DC: Author; 1999.
13. Kirkpatrick J, Richardson C, Schmeiser D, et al. Building a case for promotion of clinical faculty. Nurse Educ 2001;26(4):178–81.
14. Rice RE. Toward a broader conception of scholarship: the American context. In: Whitson TG, Geiger RL, editors. Research Universities: the United Kingdom and the United States. Buckingham (England): SRHE and the Open University; 1992. p. 117–29.
15. Mundinger MO. Clinical scholarship: DNPs add clarity. Clin Sch Rev 2009;2(1):3–4.
16. Diers D. Clinical scholarship. J Prof Nurs 1995;11(1):24–30.
17. Palmer IS. The emergence of clinical scholarship as a professional imperative. J Prof Nurs 1986;2:318–25.
18. Braxton J, Luckey W, Helland P. Institutionalizing a broader view of scholarship through Boyer's four domains. ASHE-ERIC Higher Education Report 2002;29(2): 27–33.
19. Nightingale F. Notes on nursing. London: Harrison; 1859.
20. Benner P. Uncovering the knowledge embedded in clinical practice. Image J Nurs Sch 1983;15(2):36–41.
21. Sigma Theta Tau International. Clinical scholarship resource paper. Indianapolis (IN): Author; 1999.

22. Dreher MC. Clinical scholarship: nursing practice as an intellectual endeavor. In: Clinical scholarship resource paper. Indianapolis (IN): Sigma Theta Tau International; 1999. p. 28–33.

23. National Organization of Nurse Practitioner Faculties. Faculty practice and promotion and tenure. Washington, DC: Author; 2000.

24. Blair K, Dennehy P, White P. Nurse practitioner faculty practice: an expectation of professionalism. Washington, DC: National Organization of Nurse Practitioner Faculties; 2005.

25. American Association of Colleges of Nursing. AACN position statement on the practice doctorate in nursing. Washington, DC: Author; 2004.

26. Kutzin J. Other lessons learned completing a DNP program. J Nurs Educ 2010; 39(4):181–2.

27. Institute of Medicine. The future of nursing: leading change, advancing health. Washington, DC: National Academies Press; 2011.

28. Fulton JS, Lyon BL. The need for some sense making: doctor of nursing practice. Online J Issues Nurs 2005;10(3):4.

29. Benner PE, Sutphen M, Leonard V, et al. Educating nurses: a call for radical transformation. Stanford (CA): Jossey-Bass/Carnegie Foundation for the Advancement of Teaching; 2010.

30. Danzey IM, Ea E, Fitzpatrick JJ, et al. The doctor of nursing practice and nursing education; highlights, potential and promise. J Prof Nurs 2011;27(5):311–4.

31. American Association of Colleges of Nursing. Position statement on the practice doctorate in nursing. 2004. Available at: www.aacn.nche.edu/dnp/pdf/conf/Regionals/DNPPS.pdf. Accessed April 12, 2012.

32. Kaplan L, Brown MA. Doctor of nursing practice program evaluation and beyond: capturing the profession's transition to the DNP. Nurs Educ Perspect 2009;30(6): 362–6.

33. Edwardson SR. Doctor of philosophy and doctor of nursing practice as complementary degrees. J Prof Nurs 2010;26(3):137–40.

34. Vincent D, Johnson C, Velasquez D, et al. DNP-prepared nurses as practitioner-researchers: closing the gap between research and practice. Am J Nurs Pract 2010;14(11–12):28–30, 32–4.

35. Clinton P, Sperhac AM. The DNP and unintended consequences: an opportunity for dialogue. J Pediatr Health Care 2009;23(5):348–51.

Promoting a Healthy Workplace for Nursing Faculty and Staff

Dorrie K. Fontaine, RN, PhD*, Elyta H. Koh, MBA,
Theresa Carroll, PhD

KEYWORDS

- Healthy work environments • Healthy workplace • Academia • Incivility
- Appreciative inquiry • Faculty • Staff • Schools of nursing

KEY POINTS

- Promoting a healthy workplace in academic nursing settings is vital to recruit new faculty and enhance the work life of all faculty and staff for retention and happiness.
- This article addresses the imperative of a healthy workplace, with practical suggestions for making the academic setting in schools of nursing one of optimism and confidence where future generations of nurse leaders are developed.

A leader can be a big factor in a healthy work environment, but a work environment belongs to everyone.

—E. Rudy[1(p409)]

INTRODUCTION

The campaign to focus on creating healthy work environments in clinical settings to recruit and retain nurses is nearly a decade old.[2] However, schools of nursing face a crisis of great proportion in the first decades of the twenty-first century and may require similar attention. Enormous need for new nurses educated at the highest levels coupled with a dire shortage of nursing faculty and clinical sites has created a perfect storm. This is an important time to focus on environments not only where nurses practice but also on the education arena itself, which is where the formation of the next generation of nurses occurs. Consider that when a culture of incivility is allowed to grow, it can harm the productivity and the happiness of all involved. This article

Disclosures: None of the authors has a relationship with a commercial company that has a direct financial interest in the subject matter or materials discussed in the article.
School of Nursing, University of Virginia, 225 Jeanette Lancaster Way, Charlottesville, VA 22908, USA
* Corresponding author.
E-mail address: dkf2u@virginia.edu

highlights the importance of promoting a healthy environment in academic schools of nursing where all can flourish: faculty, staff, and students. Exemplars from the University of Virginia School of Nursing are used to show one process on the journey to promoting a healthy work environment. Now is the right time to focus on the academy and a healthy workplace. With soaring retirements, new faculty and staff are all craving a supportive, even happier work environment.

NEED FOR NURSES

Schools of nursing that educate twenty-first century nurses are increasingly in the spotlight. The Bureau of Labor Statistics projects that the need for nurses will reach 1.2 million new and replacements by 2020.[3] The Future of Nursing report from the Institute of Medicine in 2010, cited the requirement for nurses to have higher levels of education, including more bachelor of science in nursing degrees, nurse practitioners, and doctorally prepared individuals.[4] The mantra of "80 by 20" is being taken as a mandate to encourage 80% of the nursing workforce to become baccalaureate prepared by 2020. It is widely acknowledged that a better-educated workforce decreases patient mortality and morbidity. All the signs point to a need for increased numbers of faculty who can teach students and meet the demand for the future workforce. The fact that 75 000 qualified applicants to schools of nursing remain on waiting lists in 2012 is a challenge to the current system.[5]

FACULTY SHORTAGES

Studies show that many schools would educate more students if the resources were there (primarily faculty and clinical sites). The American Association of Colleges of Nursing routinely estimates the growing shortage and faculty vacancies caused by insufficient funds to hire new faculty, the inability to recruit because of marketplace competition, and faculty retirements.[6] The average age of faculty is in the high 50s and growing. Creative avenues to encourage more nurses to consider a doctorate and a faculty role have been reported, such as generous foundation funding for master's graduates to go back to school[7] (eg, Jonas Center for Nursing Excellence http://www.jonascenter.org/). Encouraging nurses to consider a doctoral degree and become a faculty member is often a tough sell because of the higher salaries offered in the clinical arena, up to 25% to 30% more for nurse practitioners. It is hoped that calls for beginning doctoral study earlier in a nurse's career are making a dent. The average number of doctor of philosophy students enrolling has increased in the last 5 years (from 2007–2012) by 250 students per year, with graduations also increasing.[5] However, the question remains: Will this be enough to fill the hundreds of nursing schools seeking faculty, not to mention the diversity desired with more ethnic minorities and men? This question brings up a key dilemma: Many nursing students watch the life lived by some faculty who seem too busy, overworked, judgmental, and seemingly without joy and they reject it. The thesis of this article is that if we provided a better environment, to allow more meaningful work, and maybe even more competitive salaries, perhaps the faculty shortage would ease. There is much to be done to create healthier workplaces in academia, although little is written about this topic.

NEED FOR BALANCE

Faculty are struggling with finding balance in their life. Reports on faculty cite great stress and burnout caused by high job expectations for combining teaching, research, and service. Heavy workloads often preclude having a meaningful life outside of work.

Pressures to maintain clinical competence are high, and frustrations emerge with demands from multiple constituencies.[8] When expectations seem unrealistic, faculty can become depressed or even become hostile toward other faculty, staff, students, and administrators.[1] McBride[9] advocates for a positive mental outlook and optimism for nurse leaders, despite the chaos, and has been encouraging sustaining optimism throughout a career for nearly 20 years. She offers multiple practical tips in her book, *The Growth and Development of Nurse Leaders*, including how to understand yourself to better care for others, the appropriate use of power, handling anger, and other strategies to be successful and create more positive environments.

UNHEALTHY ENVIRONMENTS: THE PROBLEM OF INCIVILITY

Ganske[10] contends moral distress exists in academia just as it does in the clinical arena when faculty mistreat each other as well as staff and students. Although not studied in any rigorous way as yet, anecdotal evidence suggests incivility may be present and that conflict-resolution skills within a culture of trust, respect, and integrity are needed. According to Pearson and Porath,[11] in *The Cost of Bad Behavior*, incivility costs the workplace enormous damage emotionally, physically, and financially. They define incivility as "the seemingly inconsequential inconsiderate words and deeds that violate conventional norms of workplace conduct."[11] Incivility promotes negative emotions and destructive feelings. Consider these facts: 80% think incivility is a problem, 96% have experienced incivility at work, and 60% experience stress because of workplace incivility. The annual reported cost of job stress to US corporations is $300 billion.[11] **Box 1** identifies 28 examples of incivility from these researchers. Several examples may seem surprising in their subtlety, but consider how they could create a hostile environment for faculty and staff over time. Cultures that have no consequences for incivility will only further erode a respectful and healthy workplace or prevent one from ever becoming a reality.

UNHEALTHY ENVIRONMENTS: INSISTENT INDIVIDUALISM

The concept of insistent individualism may assist in explaining a perverse academic life whereby one faculty member perceives the reward structure is all about them and his or her scholarly research and does not readily volunteer for service or even for teaching students.[12] A hallmark of the behavior is not focusing on the common good. Universities may be culprits in this because they elevate competition for faculty members who have positions, tenure, and promotion to secure. An unhealthy environment is nurtured when a lack of mentoring in positive ways creates an everyone-for-oneself culture. If this sounds too severe, take a look at one or more members in each department in an academic setting and you may find them lurking, creating disloyalty, refusing assignments, and insisting that their own scholarship should take priority with or without funding. Isolation and loneliness results. If positive mentors are not on hand to orient junior faculty, is it any surprise that transgressions against fellow faculty, staff, and students can perpetuate?

Hospitality is an intriguing notion offered by Bennett.[12] He thinks the antidote to insistent individualism is a new spirit of what he refers to as *hospitality*, which features conversation as its hallmark. What should the conversation entail? The metaphor of conversation creates connectedness and accountability of all faculty for the institution as a whole. He proposes that people with different intellectual interests and histories have important things to share with each other. Students become colleagues in this metaphor as well as staff. Hospitality is an invitation to become better, per Bennett, and he advocates not only to cultivate it but also to practice it.

Box 1
Twenty-eight examples of workplace incivility

Interrupting a conversation

Checking e-mail or texting messages during a meeting

Talking loudly in common areas

Not introducing a newcomer

Failure to return a phone call

Showing little interest in another individual's opinion

Taking credit for others' efforts

Passing blame for our own mistakes

Sending bad news through e-mail so we do not have to face the recipient

Talking down to others

Not listening

Spreading rumors about colleagues

Setting others up for failure

Not saying please or thank you

Showing up late or leaving a meeting early with no explanation

Belittling others' efforts

Leaving snippy voice mail messages

Forwarding others' e-mail to make them look bad

Making demeaning or derogatory remarks to someone

Withholding information

Leaving a mess for others to clean up

Consistently grabbing easy tasks while leaving difficult ones for others

Shutting someone out of a network or team

Paying little attention or showing little interest in others' opinions

Acting irritated when someone asks for a favor

Avoiding someone

Taking resources that someone else needs

Throwing temper tantrums

From Pearson C, Porath C. The cost of bad behavior: how incivility is damaging your business and what to do about it. New York: Penguin Group; 2009; with permission.

HEALTHY WORK ENVIRONMENT STANDARDS: FROM CLINICAL TO ACADEMIC SETTINGS

A healthy, positive workplace can leverage productivity.[1] The American Association of Critical Care Nurses (AACN) developed standards for a healthy work environment in 2005 to focus on retaining nurses at the bedside to optimize their contributions and improve patient care. The 6 standards are not unique to critical care or acute care settings and actually can translate well to the business world and academia. These standards include effective communication, true collaboration, effective decision making, appropriate staffing, meaningful recognition, and authentic leadership. The clinical standards have demonstrated value in assisting nurse leaders in acute care settings to transform the workplace into one where retention is enhanced and patient outcomes are improved. **Table 1** adapts the AACN Healthy Work Environment standards for academic settings and is offered as one way to start the conversation with faculty and staff.

EXEMPLARS OF ONE JOURNEY TO A HEALTHY WORK ENVIRONMENT

A positive work environment impacts everyone. For this reason, all staff members are included in many healthy-work-environment initiatives at the University of Virginia School (UVA) of Nursing. UVA has an Appreciative Practice Center (http://www.medicine.virginia.edu/community-service/more/appreciative-practice/appreciative-practice.html). The center was created jointly by the UVA's School of Medicine, School of Nursing, Medical Center, and the physician practice plan. The purpose was to build a collaborative culture that is moving as one. Multiple projects across the university and health system demonstrate the power of this approach. The center published a book in 2011,

Table 1
Comparison of clinical and proposed academic healthy work environment standards

Standard	Clinical Setting	Proposed for Academic Setting
Communication	Nurses must be as proficient in communication skills as they are in clinical skills.	Faculty must be as proficient in communication skills as they are in teaching/clinical/research skills.
Collaboration	Nurses must be relentless in pursuing and fostering true collaboration.	Faculty must be relentless in pursuing and fostering collaboration within and beyond the university.
Effective Decision Making	Nurses must be valued and committed partners in making policy, directing and evaluating clinical care, and leading organizational operations.	Faculty must be valued and committed partners in implementing shared governance within the school and university setting.
Appropriate Staffing	Staffing must ensure the effective match between patient needs and nurse competencies.	Faculty staffing must ensure the effective match between the mission of the school and faculty competencies.
Meaningful Recognition	Nurses must be recognized and must recognize others for the value each brings to the work of the organization.	Faculty must be recognized and must recognize others for the value each brings to the work of the organization.
Authentic Leadership	Nurse leaders must fully embrace the imperative of a healthy work environment, authentically live it, and engage others in its achievement.	Faculty leaders must fully embrace the imperative of a healthy work environment, authentically live it, and engage others in its achievement.

Adapted from American Association of Critical-Care Nurses. AACN Standards for a Healthy Work Environment. Aliso Viejo (CA): AACN; 2005.

Appreciative Inquiry in Health care: Positive Questions to Bring out the Best,[13] which is an encyclopedia designed to guide other groups through the positive change process.

A new dean of the school of nursing (DKF) was appointed in 2008 who initiated a vision and focus on creating and sustaining a healthy work environment, encouraging interprofessional collaborations, and improving the diversity of faculty, staff, and students. To this end, appreciative inquiry (AI) was embraced as a philosophy and strategy, a strategic planning summit was held using AI, and a resilience room with free yoga, meditation, and mindfulness programs was created. In addition, staff members through the Administration Team were involved in defining what a healthy work environment truly means. The staff at the Office of Student and Academic Affairs was actively engaged in using AI with each other as a foundation to promote the optimal development of students in terms of body, mind, and spirit. In addition, a university-wide initiative to create a respectful workplace culminated in a new philosophy and policies. (see Respect@UVA http://www.hr.virginia.edu/other-hr-services/respectatUVa). A few highlights of these efforts are described here.

Appreciative Inquiry Summit for Strategic Planning

The AI summit was used as a method of strategic planning. Harmon and colleagues[14] published the UVA School of Nursing 2009 experience. They noted that the summit methodology using AI is not new but had not been typically used in schools of nursing. The 4-step process of discovering, dreaming, designing, and creating the school's future involved a 2-day retreat where all faculty, staff, and community stakeholders showed up to contribute. Using a model of respectful dialogue and asking positive questions, the members created the foundation of a strategic plan that was approved by all faculty and staff a year later.

The strategic plan has 3 goals and the third focuses on a healthy workplace:

Foster well being and collegial spirit in a healthy work environment (UVA School of Nursing Strategic Plan 2010–2015). Some of the strategies for meeting this goal include the following:

- Celebrate the accomplishments of all through appreciative practices in an atmosphere of collegiality, respect, and inclusion.
- Foster employee health, resilience, and well-being by offering self-care and physical activity programs, lifelong learning, and social opportunities.
- Provide healthy work, classroom, and gathering spaces.
- Enhance communication by using innovative technologies.
- Reward the accomplishments of faculty and staff through incentives, awards, bonuses. and sabbatical leaves.

The faculty members are currently working on activating the plan and implementing strategies to foster a healthy work environment in inclusive ways. Bennett's solution to promote healthier environments was to encourage conversation. This conversation is happening in intentional ways.

Using AI to Foster a Healthy Work Environment in a Student Affairs Office

The assistant dean for academic and student services (TC) continues to use the tenets of AI with all staff in the Office of Admissions and Student Services (OASS) with good results. Students report feeling exceptionally well taken care of, and staff are supported to be their best. The functional areas in a student affairs office naturally overlap and collaborate on a regular basis with each other, with students, with faculty, other administrators with the school, and many offices around the college or university. AI is a natural vehicle to use to support the 6 standards of a healthy work environment within a student affairs team.

The student affairs team has used AI to develop goals at an annual retreat, to learn how to work better together using AI interviews, and to recognize and celebrate the ways each team member depends on each other while developing authentic relationships on a daily basis.

Using AI to set team goals, OASS was able to provide staff members with an opportunity to discuss the good things done as a team. It provided a comfortable way to begin those important conversations and developed the relationships and communication necessary for a busy team with wide-ranging responsibilities to come together and build the dream for the coming year. AI's positive approach to decision making provided the staff a way to effectively evaluate programs and philosophies, create policy, and improve operations.

Even the most effective team has its bumps along the road. The AI interview technique provides leaders a way to focus on a specific issue that the staff may be having, using the *starting point questions* to discuss problems and seek answers. Whether the staff is having communication problems or cannot seem to focus on a shared goal, AI interview questions can provide a way for everyone on the team to share with others their concerns in a nonthreatening manner that leads to results.

Meaningful recognition is a core element in AI practice and a hallmark of a healthy work environment. Beginning weekly staff meetings with an appreciative moment sets a positive tone, not only for that particular hour of time but also for creating the work culture norm advocated by the Healthy Work Environment (HWE). It is easy to become consumed with the details of completing the course schedule for the next semester, awarding financial aid, arranging catering for the next event, or resolving a concern about a student. Student affairs offices are not 9-to-5 operations. There are evening workshops, weekend admissions programs, and activities and events running day in and day out. Taking the time to recognize the commitment of staff who sometimes feel like they have around-the-clock responsibilities is important, not only to create and maintain a healthy work environment but also to have fun and savor the opportunity to make a difference in someone else's life.

Case Study: Staff Involvement in Establishing a Healthy Work Environment

The engine that runs the academic mission in a university setting is the staff. Often they may be the employees with the greatest longevity and deepest loyalty. The staff members at the UVA School of Nursing have been instrumental in defining a healthy work environment, designing a tool to gather data from their colleagues, and writing a report presented to academic administrators. The following case study describes the staff's work on the healthy work environment journey through the eyes of the Associate Dean for Administration (EHK):

What does "healthy work environment" mean to you? What makes a workplace "healthy"? Is it about physical aspects such as clean air and comfortable furnishings? Are we talking about constructive relationships and respect? "Healthy work environment" is a catch phrase that conveniently encompasses all the values we uphold as ideals. It's easy to say that we believe in and want a healthy work environment, but how do we know we have one if we can't say exactly what one is? This is where the University of Virginia School of Nursing's Administration Team (all staff, ie, non-teaching and non-research employees) found themselves in the spring of 2011.

The ideal of a healthy work environment is a core value of Dean Dorrie Fontaine. She is remembered for talking about a healthy work environment during her interviews that preceded her arrival at the School of Nursing in August 2008. Before her first day, the faculty and staff were familiar with the oft repeated refrain of "healthy work environment." In October 2009, the School of Nursing conducted a two-day appreciative inquiry summit to develop a five-year strategic plan (described above).

Staff focused on the strategic initiative of a healthy work environment. While the idea resonated with them, they questioned what it really meant to their day-to-day working lives. The idea was a fuzzy notion of something positive for our work lives, but there was a growing sense that "healthy work environment" were merely words. Was there meaning, something of real value, in the words? What did the words mean? What did we want the words to mean? Were we practicing "healthy" behaviors? If not, what kind of working conditions did we have? These were common questions that came up every time "healthy work environment" was said.

After personally being asked these questions multiple times, I realized that we needed to bring meaning to these words if we truly believed in the idea and wanted it to be tangible to faculty, staff, and students. I brought together two staff members who had approached me with their questions about a healthy work environment and we deliberated ways to advance the idea. I felt strongly about two things in establishing a Healthy Work Environment (HWE) initiative: (1) the process of defining, measuring, communicating, and advancing a healthy work environment would need to be driven by stakeholders; and (2) the School of Nursing staff should take the lead in working through this process first, before expanding the initiative to the faculty and students.

I encouraged the initial two staff leaders and then the subsequent working committee to chart their own process and activities, and to present recommendations to the Dean's Council. I served as an advisor, providing ideas and suggestions along the way. The HWE working committee coordinated involvement and input of the larger Administration Team and was conscientious about being inclusive of all team members. There were several reasons to begin the HWE initiative within the Administration Team:

- Staff members are highly affected by the organizational norms and behaviors since their day-to-day work is concentrated at the School.
- Staff members likely have unique views on a healthy work environment given the relationship dynamic between faculty and staff.
- There was a desire to give staff a strong, clear voice, one that was not mixed with or influenced by faculty.
- The Administration Team could have the opportunity to lead an important school-wide initiative.

Because of these reasons, the Administration Team, led by their HWE working committee, took a central role in establishing the School of Nursing's Healthy Work Environment.

It was clear that the starting point was a definition of "healthy work environment." We needed to establish a shared meaning and an ideal to strive for. At the monthly Administration Team meeting in March 2011, the two staff leaders facilitated several brainstorming exercises with 21 participants. The first exercise asked each person to identify three key characteristics of a healthy work environment, while the second exercise asked small groups to complete the phrase, "In a healthy work environment…" Additionally, interested staff members were asked to volunteer to form a working group to advance the project, and a committee of six was established. The committee took the individual and group statements, discussed and processed the ideas, and drafted a Healthy Work Environment statement. This "compiled wisdom" was shared at the April 2011 Administration Team meeting for comments and discussion, and the final statement was accepted at the June 2011 Administration Team meeting.

Now that the Administration Team had a shared definition of a healthy work environment, the working committee moved on to the question of how the ideals translate into day-to-day actions and behaviors. How do you measure the ideals of a healthy work environment? Further, the committee pressed into the challenge of not only identifying measurable goals, but also prioritizing these ideals and evaluating the current state – answering the questions of (1) where we are now and (2) where do we want to be with respect to our healthy work environment ideal. What are our strengths and our gaps? Where do we need to focus our efforts? Over the summer and fall of 2011, the committee developed a list of measures that reflected the shared vision and definition of a healthy work environment and constructed a survey to gather both quantitative and qualitative input from the Administration Team.

The survey findings and data were provided to the Administration Team for reflection and, in December 2011, the team gathered to discuss their reactions. At this time, the Administration Team and working committee were asked to reaffirm their commitment to the HWE initiative. It was critical that the stakeholders were invested in the effort and believed in the importance of the project. The team agreed to work on and, to keep on task, the Administration Team established a timeline culminating in a presentation to the Dean's Council at the end of the spring term.

Discussion and processing of the survey results continued at a meeting in February 2012. The focus of this meeting was to talk through norms, behaviors, and characteristics for a healthy work environment. Sub-committees for each were formed to identify standards of behavior for a healthy work environment. The sub-committees synthesized and refined the behavioral expectations expressed by the Administration Team and identified short, medium, and long-term goals. The draft document for the Dean's Council was presented to and approved by the Administration Team in April.

The Healthy Work Environment working committee presented the project rationale, history, accomplishments, and recommendations to the School of Nursing Dean's Council in May 2012. The next step included inviting the faculty to join the staff in crafting strategies to encompass the School as a whole. Faculty champions have agreed and the dialog continues. The outcomes of a more engaged, respectful, and productive workplace are within our grasp.

RECOMMENDATIONS TO PROMOTE A HEALTHY WORKPLACE

Several recommendations to promote a healthy workplace are important to consider. First, an assessment of the current culture, attitudes, and values is a crucial step. Using the adapted standards for faculty as listed in **Table 1**, start a dialogue with faculty and staff on how well the workplace meets these standards. Investigate appreciative inquiry as one method to encourage a spirit of optimism and showcase strengths. Identify and cultivate faculty and staff champions who can lead the effort to a healthy workplace. Hire individuals who have a philosophy well aligned with any respectful workplace initiatives. Mentor new individuals to feel welcomed and supported. Identify any incivility wherever it occurs and address it early with consequences for poor behavior. Even better, celebrate in very visible ways when individuals act for the common good and go above and beyond. Do not be afraid to include staff with faculty in a meaningful engagement. A healthy workplace can only be achieved through dialogue and living the values an institution espouses.

SUMMARY

Promoting a healthy workplace in academic nursing settings is vital to recruit new faculty and enhance the work life of all faculty and staff for retention and happiness. Renewed attention is needed to focus on the importance of adopting standards to combat incivility, to stay optimistic despite challenges, and use the tenets of appreciative inquiry. Engaging all in crafting a culture to transform current environments is worth the effort. Only when one can unequivocally point to healthy work environments in academia will faculty embrace the lifestyle, staff find more satisfaction and meaning in their work, and students and nursing practice and discovery can flourish.

REFERENCES

1. Rudy E. Supportive work environments for nursing faculty. AACN Clin Issues 2001;12:401–10.
2. AACN standards for establishing and sustaining healthy work environments: a journey to excellence. Available at: http://www.aacn.org/WD/HWE/Docs/HWEStandards.pdf. Accessed June 17, 2012.
3. Bureau of Labor Statistics. The 30 occupations with the largest projected employment growth, 2010-20. Available at: http://www.bls.gov/news.release/ecopro.t06.htm. Accessed June 17, 2012.
4. IOM (Institute of Medicine). The future of nursing: leading change, advancing health. Washington, DC: The National Academies Press; 2010.
5. Fang D, Li Y, Bednash GD. 2011–2012 Enrollment and graduations in baccalaureate and graduate programs in nursing. Washington, DC: American Association of Colleges of Nursing; 2012.
6. Fang D, Li Y. Special survey on vacant faculty positions for academic year 2011-2012. 2012. Available at: http://www.aacn.nche.edu/leading-initiatives/research-data/vacancy11.pdf. Accessed June 17, 2012.
7. Fontaine DK, Dracup K. The accelerated doctoral program in nursing: a university-foundation partnership. J Nurs Educ 2007;46:159–64.
8. Shirey MR. Stress and burnout in nursing faculty. Nurse Educ 2006;31:95–7.
9. McBride AB. The growth and development of nurse leaders. New York: Springer Publishing Company; 2011.
10. Ganske KM. Moral distress in academia. Online J Issues Nurs 2010;15(3). Manuscript 6.
11. Pearson C, Porath C. The cost of bad behavior: how incivility is damaging your business and what to do about it. New York: Penguin Group; 2009.
12. Bennett JB. Academic life: hospitality, ethics, and spirituality. Boston: Anker Publishing; 2003.
13. May N, Becker D, Frankel R, et al. Appreciative inquiry in healthcare: positive questions to bring out the best. Brunswick (OH): Crown Publishing Company; 2011.
14. Harmon RH, Fontaine D, Plews-Ogan M, et al. Achieving transformational change: using appreciative inquiry for strategic planning in a school of nursing. J Prof Nurs 2012;28:119–24.

The Experience of a New Deanship for Two Robert Wood Johnson Foundation Executive Nurse Fellows

Rosalie O. Mainous, PhD, APRN, NNP-BC[a,*],
Stephen J. Cavanagh, PhD, MPA, RN, FRSPH, FinstLM[b]

KEYWORDS

- Dean • Transitions • Leadership • Strategic planning • Personnel management
- Robert Wood Johnson Foundation

KEY POINTS

- Take time to assess and resist the temptation to change without understanding.
- Build your team; look to engage and reinvigorate faculty and staff.
- Negotiate, demonstrate, and communicate the vision for the future.
- When leading, be consistent and transparent.

So, you have been through the dean interviews, met with the faculty, communicated with administrators and other constituents, and presented your vision for the future. You are offered the job of the next dean of nursing. Fortified with a sense of having entered into a social contract with faculty and armed with a charter for action, what do you do? Well, for the first few weeks, at least, perhaps nothing, at least nothing transformational.

BACKGROUND

What does a dean do? The role in the early part of the twentieth century involved student issues; today's deans are responsible for the budget, personnel issues, fundraising, oversight of the curriculum in light of resources, and, more recently, entrepreneurship.[1]

Disclosures: None of the authors has a relationship with a commercial company that has a direct financial interest in the subject matter or materials discussed in the article.
[a] Miami Valley College of Nursing and Health, Wright State University, 160 University Hall, 3640 Colonel Glenn Highway, Dayton, OH 45435, USA; [b] School of Nursing, University of Massachusetts Amherst, 651 North Pleasant Street, Amherst, MA 01003-9299, USA
* Corresponding author.
E-mail address: Rosalie.mainous@wright.edu

For a dean new to an organization, some have argued that there are predictable phases to the role of dean.[2] These have been characterized as honeymoon, disenchantment, reality, maturity, and a golden phase.[3] From the perspective of a new dean, the idea of a honeymoon period may be characterized by individual excitement and enthusiasm at being able to work with new people to fulfill individual, faculty, and institutional goals. Although these early weeks and months are a time of understanding the organization and fostering new relationships, the dean must also demonstrate political and business acumen; this is the time to negotiate the resources essential for a college to achieve its mission and goals. There are other perspectives on the honeymoon period. For one, the period provides an opportunity for assessing a new organization and its strengths and weaknesses and offers a new dean time for thoughtful reflection without necessarily being required to act and institute change immediately. But it can also be a period where there are opportunities for a new dean to be forgiven for not immediately understanding the inner workings and acting in ways that might seem to be out of character with the organizational culture. In either case, Watkins[4] acknowledges that the first 3 months of a new appointment can be highly influential in the development of the relationship between leader, faculty, and staff. The honeymoon period may also be characterized as a time when the newly appointed dean's efforts are centered on short-term issues, building relationships, and leading an organization's activities.

ASSESSMENT STAGE

From a personal perspective, the first 90 days of a deanship also has phases, critical activities that are essential to negotiate successfully if the dean is to achieve the organizational mission and goals. The first of these might be considered the assessment stage. There is inevitably a great temptation to rush into action and bring about organizational change, given that your appointment was predicated on a vision that was seen as important and coherent with the organization. During these early days, it is important to assess the organization and, if necessary, be prepared to do nothing, but all the time listening and observing. Although it is tempting to quickly become the architect of a well-constructed organizational plan, this cannot be done effectively without understanding what you have inherited.[5] The dean must understand how things work before attempting to change things. This is important because progress toward new goals requires leadership and change. For this to be effective, there has to be a separation from the past—the old ways that may no longer be effective in the current educational or business climate.[6] At the same time, an organization's history is important to avoid a déjà vu climate, where there is reinventing of the same mistakes or inefficiencies of the past without a clear rationale and justification. Nevertheless, a new dean has to make an honest and balanced assessment quickly and find a balance between introspection and acting circumspectly and the importance of changing what is not working. This is crucial given that part of a new leader's role is to overcome institution and faculty inertia and create a momentum to achieve new goals and expectations. During this assessment phase, a dean is going to find issues and problems that need a solution. Without a thorough assessment, a dean must resist the temptation to answer questions too soon without fully understanding the complexity and nuances of what this means.

During this early assessment, it is highly likely that there are problems not disclosed when negotiating the initial appointment contract. Some may only be known by those in the college; others may be well known by the president and provost as well as the community at large. Spend the first 6 to 9 months taking care of critical issues that may involve public relations, curricular change, organizational culture, National Council

Licensure Examination scores, and faculty turnover. These internal reviews are essential because they may identify areas that need immediate attention. Failure to identify or manage these college friction points may jeopardize your credibility and ability to move forward with a new agenda. Resolving such issues at home is important to allow issues that are external to the college to be addressed. A modern dean of nursing must also show leadership in the areas of alumni relations, development, community collaborations, and new program development while demonstrating an ability to cultivate political confidences.

A new dean must develop new ways of thinking. Put people first[7] and recognize that deans cannot be a success alone. Approximately one-fifth of all deanships in the nation turn over every year due to factors, such as attrition, retirement, or movement up the career ladder.[1] Not all deans are a good fit, however, even with the careful selection process most universities have in place. Some of them move out of the position, some drop into a faculty line, and some seek employment elsewhere. Listen to the messages received from the provost or chancellor. Are you expected to be a scholar? A fundraiser? A manager? It is projected that a successful transition process as a new dean can take from 18 to 30 months.

TEAM BUILDING

As a new dean, it is important to build a team of faculty and staff in whom you have confidence. Early on, assess senior faculty who have administrative or functional roles, not necessarily in the obvious ways of being expert educators or administrators, although these are essential qualities. Do they understand and are they able to convey the vision you are espousing? It is also important to look for the knowledge and skills needed to educate tomorrow's nurses and those capable of enabling the future of health care and the development of the profession. At the same time, it is inevitable that efforts will be necessary to invigorate and re-engage faculty and staff toward activities important to the organization. The importance of visibility to faculty and staff cannot be overestimated. Meet with all employees one-on-one, participate in faculty and staff events, engage in routine conversations, and manage by walking around. When interacting with faculty and staff, know your strengths and assets. Change requires energy, commitment, and knowledge to overcome organizational inertia and to answer critics who may ask, Why this change and why now?

NEGOTIATING THE VISION

An essential component of a new dean's role is to negotiate the social mandate for change. What this involves is a process whereby expectations are discussed, clarified, and agreed on. Successful negotiation requires a visualization, simulation, or definition of what achievement or success looks like. Plans, which should be in writing, must also include ways to manage expectations. Part of this process is to ask faculty to answer key questions, for example, Who are we as a school? This questioning is important because it sets the tone for the organizational activities, such as new appointments, resource expenditures, and where to invest effort.

For a new dean, there are great opportunities to successfully manage this process and, at the same time, dangers. Deans should look for ways of modeling or creating the guiding vision[8] as a way to begin the momentum of change. Quick impact–quick wins may present themselves. Initiating actions (eg, small internal research grant awards) can have an immediate impact on faculty activity and morale, while at the same time providing an opportunity to demonstrate the importance of research going forward. Engage faculty early to help build and establish personal credibility and political capital, but be careful not to pressure yourself to overdeliver too soon. The goal is not to shock faculty with a new vision; sometimes when illumination and clarity of direction are all that is required, it is better to be a candle than a supernova.

Modeling a vision can be a useful way to engage faculty, staff, and the organization in new directions, priorities, and policies. This by itself may not be sufficient. Managing the communication pathways within the school and the messages is equally important. Develop ways of distributing your message to faculty and staff, seek out opportunities to develop speaking skills, and get visibility. Create opportunities to tell the leadership story. This is essential because effective leadership and change require a mobilization and commitment to the vision.[5] The litmus test of success in developing commitment is the extent to which faculty and staff members identify their actions as contributing to the vision. This request for commitment may require a dean to manage those faculty and staff members who, for whatever reason, no longer feel able to continue their careers or employment with the organization.

LEADERSHIP

Leadership competencies have been identified[9] for the next decade. Among these are the abilities to team build and demonstrate authenticity, political savvy, a global perspective, and expert decision-making skills. A leader must also be technologically competent to develop relationships. Leadership is ultimately about relationships; without the ability to communicate competently in all mediums, these relationships are at risk. Frequent communiqués from the dean's office are usually needed, particularly in the first year. One method is to send a short newsletter bimonthly explaining where you have been, partnerships being forged, and what the impact on faculty and staff may be.

Strategic planning is critical. This plan should be based on the assessment, the vision statement crafted with the faculty, and consistency with the university strategic plan. Develop a presence within the university community and become recognized in the community at large. Having a strategic plan that is also in line with the goals of clinical partners is helpful. The college cannot be all things to all people, however. Carefully and strategically identify areas of action. Be wary of falling into the trap of constantly referring back to your previous institution as an example. This grows old quickly and implies to the faculty that you have not yet really disconnected with your previous place of employment.

Strategic planning is essential. During the early weeks and months of a deanship, there is a natural tendency to be introspective when seeking to understand leadership issues and understanding the full extent of the resources available. During this early period, time should be taken to review the resources and expertise available on the advisory body that may exist. Members of this group can become a valuable asset to the work of a dean. As with any committee, time is well spent in understanding the workings of the board and developing a good working relationship with its chair. Opportunities should be taken to share perceptions about the school and any area of concern or challenge. Members of external advisory committees can help support the dean in understanding the local community, business, and development opportunities as well as how the school is perceived in general. Members of external boards are likely to have been the choice of the school's previous dean, and an honest assessment should be undertaken to ensure that the repertoire of talent available is in keeping with current needs. To this extent, the board may need to be re-engineered to meet new and emerging challenges that now present themselves. This may be difficult to assess in the early months of a deanship in terms of balance.

To what extent should the board membership focus on development or fundraising issues; functional skills, such as marketing and communication; or knowledge of local health care providers? The answer probably lies with a mixture of all of these. In any case, external board members should be actively engaged in supporting and advising the dean and not be perceived as ceremonial or honorary positions. A dean may be wise to review the relevant bylaws relating to the board and ensure that duties, expectations, and terms of reappointment are clearly understood and documented.

A new deanship not only implies moving from one role to another but also generally from one culture, environment, or institution to one that is new and different. Excluding internal candidates who assume a deanship, others must negotiate a new job and new territory. It may be a geographic change, Carnegie classification change, public versus private, and so on. Following are experiences of the authors.

LIVING WITH A COLLECTIVE BARGAINING AGREEMENT

Movement from an academic environment without a union to one in which a union is entrenched can be fraught with difficulties. Working with a unionized faculty involves a culture change and the need to reflect on the agreement before every decision. It is wise to become as familiar as possible with all of the nuances of the agreement. Decisions as mundane as to when a syllabus must be available to students may be dictated by a collective bargaining agreement.

Colleges bogged down in grievances and appeals have a direct impact on the academic mission and the success of the students. The usual scenario involves a faculty member and administration. Both have worthy perspectives, and both want the best outcome. Occasionally, however, the union has internal struggles—faculty to faculty. This scenario is even more disruptive than faculty versus administration. Everyone expects administration to be heavy handed. It is distressing to the faculty, however, to have to make decisions in the process of self-governance that may not be perceived as in the best interest of all. This leads to a grievance and the union finds itself advocating for one group of their constituents against other, just as loyal, union members. It is best for the dean to stay as far removed from this situation as possible while upholding appropriate processes used in the conduct of college business.

Integrity and honesty are critical.[10] In the early phases of interaction with faculty and the union representatives, it is critical that decisions are reflective of a high degree of integrity. This is not to say that when a relationship is on solid footing, one should regress. What it implies is that first impressions are everything, and it is hard to gain momentum with a union if there is an early mistake or misperception.

Transition from an Urban University to a Rural Institution

Irrespective of how much planning has gone into choosing a job, there will be some surprises. The move from an urban school with a predominantly commuter student body to a rural land-grant university with a substantial residential population is a significant change of pace. The time between meetings on campus needs careful choreography and necessitates the surrendering of the diary/calendar to a personal assistant. Due to the importance and frequency of athletic and sporting events, new-student orientations, and alumni functions, many evenings and weekend are spent on campus. In addition, having a significant alumni base in a major metropolitan area some distance from the school frequently requires up to 4 hours per day in traveling time. These types of meetings are important for new deans to participate in but require balancing the needs of internal student and faculty needs with those of external constituents and fundraising. These factors also have an impact on the questions of whether to focus early efforts on understanding the internal aspects of the school and university versus constituency building and spending time external to the school. The reality is, of course, that a balance needs to be struck between the 2 activities. This balance is influenced by the strength of the team you have built and the confidence you have in letting them perform the duties for which they are responsible. There can be the temptation to become personally involved in decision making at a microlevel or simply using your position to solve problems that are the responsibility of others. This is seldom helpful for morale or teambuilding and can foster a culture of second guessing the dean. Be clear on what the responsibilities of your team are and provide resources for them to be successful. The internal versus external debate can also be influenced by internal university policy, for example, the beginning of a capital campaign. This activity necessitates working with, informing, and mobilizing the support of alumni and the business community in development activities. This requires visibility, a strong message, and the ability to engage people in participating in the future of the school or college.

SUMMARY

There are key principles that should be embraced to move through the transition smoothly and to emerge a respected leader.

1. Put your employees first and reward them for their successes publicly. Everyone likes to be valued and acknowledged.
2. Listen carefully before rendering an opinion. The culture is different, and new rules apply.
3. Find the historian. Find out how things have been done in the past. This does not necessarily mean you must repeat the process, but knowing from whence they come is valuable.
4. Quickly ascertain who the informal leaders are and what makes them powerful. Respect their position in the institution.
5. Be fiscally conservative.
6. There should be consequences for bad behavior. Bad behaviors on the part of a few demoralize those that are working hard to do all of the right things.
7. Transparency, transparency, transparency.
8. Be yourself. You will never be able to maintain a facade, particularly in times of stress.
9. Role model for the faculty. No one likes "do as I say, not as I do."
10. Be strategic and do not get sucked in by pet projects. You will have to make hard decisions, and not everyone will like the decision. If the decision is well thought out, based on evidence, and is ethical, stand by the decision. After all, you are the dean.

The Robert Wood Johnson Foundation Executive Nurse Fellows program is a substantial investment in the future of nursing. Leadership training as an overriding theme and personal development as a subtheme are the cornerstones of success for this program. With the help of the Robert Wood Johnson Foundation, seasoned educators, hospital administrators, and leaders in public health nursing come together and learn a common language as well as acquire leadership competencies to move the nursing profession forward. It is this program, along with life leadership experiences, that enables emerging leaders to move to the forefront and to begin to make a substantial impact on the health care system.

REFERENCES

1. Wolverton M, Gmelch WH, Montez J, et al. ASHE-ERIC Higher Education Report 2001;28(1).
2. Pressler JL, Kenner C. Making the most of the "honeymoon phase" of a deanship. Nurse Educ 2008;33(1):1–3.
3. Gottman JM, Silver N. The seven principles of making a marriage work. New York: Three Rivers Press; 2000.
4. Watkins M. The first 90 days: critical success strategies for all new leaders at all levels. Boston: Harvard Business School Press; 2003.
5. Tichy NM, Devanna MA. Transformational leader: the key to global competitiveness. Hoboken (NJ): John Wiley & Sons; 1997.
6. Kanter RM, Stein BA, Jick TD. The challenge of organizational change; how companies experience it and leaders guide it. New York: Simon & Schuster; 1992.
7. Novak D. Taking people with you: the only way to make big things happen. New York: Penguin Group; 2012.
8. Kotter J. Leading change. Boston: Harvard Business School Press; 1996.
9. Huston C. Preparing nurse leaders for 2020. J Nurs Manag 2008;16(8):905–11.
10. Bassaw B. Determinants of successful deanship. Med Teach 2010;32(12): 1002–2006.

Index

Note: Page numbers of article titles are in **boldface** type.

A

Academic settings. *See* Schools of nursing.
Accelerated programs, in nursing education, 429
Affordable Care Act, paradigm shift in nursing education to comply with, **455–462**
Appreciative inquiry, as strategy for a healthy workplace, 562–563
Autism, preparing nurses to care for people with developmental disabilities, **517–527**

B

Bachelor of Science in Nursing (BSN), essential genetics/genomics competencies for, 535
    trends in BSN curricula, 537–538
Boyer's model of scholarship, 549–550
Business, incorporating Toyota Production System into nursing curricula, **503–516**

C

Cerebral palsy, preparing nurses to care for people with developmental disabilities, **517–527**
Chromosomal microarray, in assessment of genetic contribution to health and illness,
    531–532
Clinical education, of primary care nurse practitioners, **455–462**
Clinical practice, promoting a healthy workplace, **557–566**
Collaboration, interprofessional educational, effect on patient outcomes, 496–499
Collective bargaining agreements, experience of new deans with, 571–572
Competency-based education, for primary care nurse practitioner clinical education,
    455–462
Computer-based simulation, to enhance clinical judgment skills in senior nursing students,
    481–491
        data analysis and results, 486–488
        discussion, 488
        implications for experiential learning theory, 488–489
        literature on, 483–484
        methods, 484–486
Core competencies, in genetics/genomics, implementation of, 541–542
Curricula, nursing, incorporating Toyota Production System into, **503–516**
        background, 504–505
        Drexel University's journey, 508–512
            classroom incorporation of TPS, 509–510
            clinical incorporation of TPS, 510–512
            early implementation, 508–509
            incorporation of active learning strategies, 510
        recommendations, 512–513
        Toyota principles in health care, 507–508
        Toyota Production System, 505–507

Nurs Clin N Am 47 (2012) 575–582
http://dx.doi.org/10.1016/S0029-6465(12)00098-9
0029-6465/12/$ – see front matter © 2012 Elsevier Inc. All rights reserved.
nursing.theclinics.com

D

Deans, of schools of nursing, experience of new, **567–573**
    assessment stage, 568–569
    background, 567–568
    leadership, 570–571
    living with a collective bargaining agreement, 571–572
    negotiating the vision, 569–570
    team building, 569
    transition from urban university to rural institution, 571–572
Dedicated education units, in nursing education, 429
Developmental disabilities, preparing nurses to care for people with, **517–527**
    descriptive reports of educational strategies, 522–523
    education of health care providers to address gaps and disparities, 520–521
    faculty considerations, 521
    integration of concepts and experiences in, 521–522
    population considerations, 518–520
    research on educational strategies, 523
Diversity, in nursing student population, 427
Doctor of Nursing Practice (DNP) degree, graduates with, as faculty members, **547–556**
    advantages to schools of nursing employing, 553–554
    arrival of practice scholar in academic setting, 548–549
    barriers facing, 550–553
        operationalizing concept of clinical scholarship, 550–551
        promotion and tenure issues, 552–553
        relationship to clinical practice, 551–552
        role expectations for, 551
    Boyer's model of scholarship revisited, 549–550
    future of faculty composition, 554
    historical composition of faculty, 547–548
    traditional faculty roles, 547–548
national study of nursing faculty with, **435–453**
    background, 436–437
    discussion, 446–450
    implications, 450–452
        faculty recruitment and retention, 450–451
        impact of DNP, 451
        next generation of faculty, 451
        research and scholarship of DNP, 451
        succession planning, 450
        trends in tenure, 451–452
    methodology, 438–439
    results, 439–446
        comparisons between PhD and DNP faculty, 443–445
        DNP and PhD, 439–441
        nursing faculty in doctoral education, 441–442
        professional growth and work satisfaction, 442
        professional profile of participants, 439
        qualitative comments, 445–446
        succession planning and future vision, 443

Doctor of Philosophy (PhD) in Nursing, in national study of doctoral nursing faculty, **435–453**
  comparison with DNP degree, 439–441, 443–445
Drexel University, interprofessional education collaboration at, 499–500

E

Education, nursing. *See* Nursing education.
Experiential learning theory, impact of computer-based simulation on, 488–489

F

Faculty, Doctor of Nursing Practice (DNP) graduates as, **547–556**
  advantages to schools of nursing employing, 553–554
  arrival of practice scholar in academic setting, 548–549
  barriers facing, 550–553
    operationalizing concept of clinical scholarship, 550–551
    promotion and tenure issues, 552–553
    relationship to clinical practice, 551–552
    role expectations for, 551
  Boyer's model of scholarship revisited, 549–550
  future of composition of, 554
  historical composition of, 547–548
  traditional roles, 547–548
  national survey of doctoral nursing, **435–453**
  promoting a healthy workplace for, **557–566**
  shortages of, 558

G

Genetics, call for research on, in nursing education, **529–545**
  genomics and, in health promotion and disease treatment, 530–532
    assessment of genetic contribution to health and illness, 531–532
    integration into clinical care, 531
    therapeutics, 532
  in popular culture and public discourse, 532–533
    early education in, 532–533
  proposed best practice needs evidence, 539–542
    genetic literacy, 539–541
    implementation of core competencies, 541–542
    recommendations, 539
  systematic training for health care providers, 533–539
    BSN essentials, 535
    current approach, 537–538
    Genetics/Genomic Competency Center for Education, 538–539
    MSN essentials, 535–537
    strategic plan, 534–535
Genetics/Genomics Competency Center for Education (G2C2), 535–536
Genomics, in nursing education. *See* Genetics.
Growth, professional, of doctoral nursing faculty, 442

H

Health care reform, and paradigm shift in nursing education, **455–462**
    impact on primary care nurse practitioner clinical education, **455–462**
Health promotion, role of genetics/genomics in, 530–532

I

Incivility, in the workplace, 559
Insistent individualism, in the workplace, 559–560
Institute of Medicine, Future of Nursing Initiative, paradigm shift in nursing education to
    comply with, **455–462**
Intellectual disabilities, preparing nurses to care for people with, **517–527**
Interprofessional education, impact on patient outcomes, 496–499

J

Judgment skills, impact of computer-based simulation on clinical, **481–491**

K

Knowledge, explosion of, in nursing education, 427
Kolb's experiential learning theory, 482–483

L

Leadership, experience of new deans, 570–571
Learner-centered environments, 424–425

M

Masters of Science in Nursing (MSN), essential genetics/genomics competencies for,
    535–537

N

Nurse Executive Fellows, of Robert Wood Johnson Foundation, experience of
    new deanship for two, **567–573**
Nurse practitioners, clinical education in primary care, **463–479**
        approach, 465
        background, 464–465
        gap analysis, 465
        literature review, 465–470
        standards for, 470–476
Nurses, need for, 558
Nursing education, 423–567
    computer-based simulation to enhance clinical judgment skills, **481–491**
        data analysis and results, 486–488
        discussion, 488
        implications for experiential learning theory, 488–489
        Kolb's experiential learning theory and, 482–483
        literature on, 483–484
        methods, 484–486

Doctor of Nursing Practice graduates as faculty member, **547–556**
 advantages to schools of nursing employing, 553–554
 arrival of practice scholars in academic setting, 548–549
 barriers facing, 550–553
 Boyer's model of scholarship revisited, 549–550
 historical composition of faculty, 557–558
 traditional faculty roles, 547–548
doctoral nursing faculty, national study of, **435–453**
 background, 436–437
 discussion, 446–450
 implications, 450–452
 methodology, 438–439
 results, 439–446
experience of new deans, **567–573**
 assessment stage, 568–569
 background, 567–568
 leadership, 570–571
 living with a collective bargaining agreement, 571–572
 negotiating the vision, 569–570
 team building, 569
 transition from urban university to rural institution, 571–572
genomic literacy and competent practice, **529–545**
 genetics and genomics in health promotion and disease treatment, 530–532
 genetics in popular culture and public discourse, 532–533
 proposed best practice needs evidence, 539–542
 systematic training for health care providers, 533–539
incorporating Toyota Production System into nursing curricula, **503–516**
 background, 504–505
 Drexel University's journey, 508–512
 recommendations, 512–513
 Toyota principles in health care, 507–508
 Toyota Production System, 505–507
on caring for people with developmental disabilities, **517–527**
 descriptive reports of educational strategies, 522–523
 education of health care providers to address gaps and disparities, 520–521
 faculty considerations, 521
 integration of concepts and experiences in, 521–522
 population considerations, 518–520
 research on educational strategies, 523
paradigm shift in, **455–462**
 case study, 457–461
primary care nurse practitioner clinical education, **463–479**
 approach, 465
 background, 464–465
 gap analysis, 465
 literature review, 465–470
 standards for, 470–476
promoting a healthy workplace for faculty and staff, **557–566**
 exemplars of one journey, 561–565
 faculty shortages, 558
 need for balance, 558–559

Nursing education (*continued*)
    need for nurses, 558
    recommendations for, 565
    standards for clinical to academic settings, 560–561
    unhealthy environments, 559–560
        incivility, 559
        insistent individualism, 559–560
  transdisciplinary simulation, **493–502**
    background and significance, 494–495
    Drexel IPEC, 499–500
    evidence that interprofessional education improves patient outcomes, 496–499
    lessons learned, 495–496
    summary and future visions, 500
  trends in, **423–434**
    accelerated programs, 428
    background and history, 423–424
    case studies, 428–429
    challenges in transforming, 430–432
    clinical immersion experiences, 429
    concepts-based curricula, 429
    dedicated education units, 429
    diverse student populations, 427
    external reports/recommendations, 425–427
    knowledge explosion, 427
    new program options, 428
    simulation, 428
    teacher centered and learner-centered environments, 424–425
    technology, 427–428
Nursing schools. *See* Schools of nursing.

O

Outcomes, evidence that interprofessional education improves patient, 496–499

P

Patient Protection and Affordable Care Act, paradigm shift in nursing education to comply with, **455–462**
Primary care, clinical education of nurse practitioners in, **463–479**
  approach, 465
  background, 464–465
  gap analysis, 465
  literature review, 465–470
  standards for, 470–476
  paradigm shift in nursing education to comply with health care reform in, **455–462**
Professional growth, of doctoral nursing faculty, 442
Promotions, of doctoral nursing faculty, 552–553

R

Recruitment, of doctoral nursing faculty, 450–451
Research, by DNP-degreed nursing faculty, 451

Retention, of doctoral nursing faculty, 450–451
Robert Wood Johnson Foundation, experience of new deanship for two Nurse Executive Fellows of, **567–573**

S

Salary, of doctoral nursing faculty, 443
Satisfaction, work, of doctoral nursing faculty, 442
Scholarship, Boyer's model of, 549–550
    clinical, operationalizing concept of, 550–551
    of DNP nursing faculty, 451
Schools of nursing, advantages of employing DNP graduates as faculty, 553–554
    experience of new deans, **567–573**
        assessment stage, 568–569
        background, 567–568
        leadership, 570–571
        living with a collective bargaining agreement, 571–572
        negotiating the vision, 569–570
        team building, 569
        transition from urban university to rural institution, 571–572
    promoting a healthy work environment in, **557–566**
        exemplars of one journey, 561–565
        faculty shortages, 558
        need for balance, 558–559
        need for nurses, 558
        recommendations for, 565
        standards for clinical to academic settings, 560–561
        unhealthy environments, 559–560
            incivility, 559
            insistent individualism, 559–560
Simulation, computer-based, to enhance clinical judgment skills, **481–491**
        data analysis and results, 486–488
        discussion, 488
        implications for experiential learning theory, 488–489
        Kolb's experiential learning theory and, 482–483
        literature on, 483–484
        methods, 484–486
    in nursing education, 429
    transdisciplinary, **493–502**
        background and significance, 494–495
        Drexel IPEC, 499–500
        evidence that interprofessional education improves patient outcomes, 496–499
        lessons learned, 495–496
        summary and future visions, 500
Staff, promoting a healthy workplace for, **557–566**
Strategic planning, experience of new deans, 569–570
Students, impact of computer-based simulation on clinical judgment skills, **481–491**
Succession planning, for doctoral nursing faculty, 443, 450

T

Teacher-centered environments, 424–425
Technology, trends in nursing education, 427–428

Tenure, of doctoral nursing faculty, 451–452, 552–553
Toyota Production System, incorporating into nursing curricula, **503–516**
    background, 504–505
    Drexel University's journey, 508–512
        classroom incorporation of TPS, 509–510
        clinical incorporation of TPS, 510–512
        early implementation, 508–509
        incorporation of active learning strategies, 510
    recommendations, 512–513
    Toyota principles in health care, 507–508
    Toyota Production System, 505–507
Transdisciplinary simulation, **493–502**
    background and significance, 494–495
    Drexel IPEC, 499–500
    evidence that interprofessional education improves patient outcomes, 496–499
    lessons learned, 495–496
    summary and future visions, 500
Transformation, of nursing education, 430–432
Transitions, experience of new deans, **567–573**
Trends, in nursing education, **423–434**
    accelerated programs, 428
    background and history, 423–424
    case studies, 428–429
    challenges in transforming, 430–432
    clinical immersion experiences, 429
    concepts-based curricula, 429
    dedicated education units, 429
    diverse student populations, 427
    external reports/recommendations, 425–427
    knowledge explosion, 427
    new program options, 428
    simulation, 428
    teacher centered and learner-centered environments, 424–425
    technology, 427–428

W

Work environment, promotion of healthy, for faculty and staff, **557–566**
    exemplars of one journey, 561–565
    faculty shortages, 558
    need for balance, 558–559
    need for nurses, 558
    recommendations for, 565
    standards for clinical to academic settings, 560–561
    unhealthy environments, 559–560
        incivility, 559
        insistent individualism, 559–560
Work satisfaction, of doctoral nursing faculty, 442

United States Postal Service

Statement of Ownership, Management, and Circulation
(All Periodicals Publications Except Requestor Publications)

1. Publication Title	2. Publication Number	3. Filing Date
Nursing Clinics of North America	5 9 8 - 9 6 0 0	9/14/12

4. Issue Frequency	5. Number of Issues Published Annually	6. Annual Subscription Price
Mar, Jun, Sep, Dec	4	$144.00

7. Complete Mailing Address of Known Office of Publication *(Not printer)* *(Street, city, county, state, and ZIP+4®)*

Elsevier Inc.
360 Park Avenue South
New York, NY 10010-1710

Contact Person
Stephen R. Bushing
Telephone *(Include area code)*
215-239-3688

8. Complete Mailing Address of Headquarters or General Business Office of Publisher *(Not printer)*

Elsevier Inc., 360 Park Avenue South, New York, NY 10010-1710

9. Full Names and Complete Mailing Addresses of Publisher, Editor, and Managing Editor *(Do not leave blank)*

Publisher *(Name and complete mailing address)*

Kim Murphy, Elsevier, Inc., 1600 John F. Kennedy Blvd. Suite 1800, Philadelphia, PA 19103-2899

Editor *(Name and complete mailing address)*

Katie Hartner, Elsevier, Inc., 1600 John F. Kennedy Blvd. Suite 1800, Philadelphia, PA 19103-2899

Managing Editor *(Name and complete mailing address)*

Adrianne Brigido, Elsevier, Inc., 1600 John F. Kennedy Blvd. Suite 1800, Philadelphia, PA 19103-2899

10. Owner *(Do not leave blank. If the publication is owned by a corporation, give the name and address of the corporation immediately followed by the names and addresses of all stockholders owning or holding 1 percent or more of the total amount of stock. If not owned by a corporation, give the names and addresses of the individual owners. If owned by a partnership or other unincorporated firm, give its name and address as well as those of each individual owner. If the publication is published by a nonprofit organization, give its name and address.)*

Full Name	Complete Mailing Address
Wholly owned subsidiary of	1600 John F. Kennedy Blvd., Ste. 1800
Reed/Elsevier, US holdings	Philadelphia, PA 19103-2899

11. Known Bondholders, Mortgagees, and Other Security Holders Owning or Holding 1 Percent or More of Total Amount of Bonds, Mortgages, or Other Securities. If none, check box ☐ None

Full Name	Complete Mailing Address
N/A	

12. Tax Status *(For completion by nonprofit organizations authorized to mail at nonprofit rates)* *(Check one)*
The purpose, function, and nonprofit status of this organization and the exempt status for federal income tax purposes:
☐ Has Not Changed During Preceding 12 Months
☐ Has Changed During Preceding 12 Months *(Publisher must submit explanation of change with this statement)*

PS Form 3526, September 2007 (Page 1 of 3 *(Instructions Page 3)*) PSN 7530-01-000-9931 PRIVACY NOTICE: See our Privacy policy in www.usps.com

---

13. Publication Title	14. Issue Date for Circulation Data Below
Nursing Clinics of North America	September 2012

15. Extent and Nature of Circulation		Average No. Copies Each Issue During Preceding 12 Months	No. Copies of Single Issue Published Nearest to Filing Date
a. Total Number of Copies *(Net press run)*		1835	1639
b. Paid Circulation (By Mail and Outside the Mail)	(1) Mailed Outside-County Paid Subscriptions Stated on PS Form 3541. *(Include paid distribution above nominal rate, advertiser's proof copies, and exchange copies)*	1163	1064
	(2) Mailed In-County Paid Subscriptions Stated on PS Form 3541 *(Include paid distribution above nominal rate, advertiser's proof copies, and exchange copies)*		
	(3) Paid Distribution Outside the Mails Including Sales Through Dealers and Carriers, Street Vendors, Counter Sales, and Other Paid Distribution Outside USPS®	291	318
	(4) Paid Distribution by Other Classes Mailed Through the USPS (e.g. First-Class Mail®)		
c. Total Paid Distribution *(Sum of 15b (1), (2), (3), and (4))*	▶	1454	1382
d. Free or Nominal Rate Distribution (By Mail and Outside the Mail)	(1) Free or Nominal Rate Outside-County Copies Included on PS Form 3541	60	67
	(2) Free or Nominal Rate In-County Copies Included on PS Form 3541		
	(3) Free or Nominal Rate Copies Mailed at Other Classes Through the USPS (e.g. First-Class Mail)		
	(4) Free or Nominal Rate Distribution Outside the Mail (Carriers or other means)		
e. Total Free or Nominal Rate Distribution *(Sum of 15d (1), (2), (3) and (4))*	▶	60	67
f. Total Distribution *(Sum of 15c and 15e)*	▶	1514	1449
g. Copies not Distributed *(See instructions to publishers #4 (page 83))*	▶	321	190
h. Total *(Sum of 15f and g)*	▶	1835	1639
i. Percent Paid (15c divided by 15f times 100)		96.04%	95.38%

16. Publication of Statement of Ownership

If the publication is a general publication, publication of this statement is required. Will be printed in the December 2012 issue of this publication. ☐ Publication not required.

17. Signature and Title of Editor, Publisher, Business Manager, or Owner

[signature] Stephen R. Bushing –Inventory/Distribution Coordinator

Date September 14, 2012

I certify that all information furnished on this form is true and complete. I understand that anyone who furnishes false or misleading information on this form or who omits material or information requested on the form may be subject to criminal sanctions (including fines and imprisonment) and/or civil sanctions (including civil penalties).

PS Form 3526, September 200 (Page 2 of 3)

Moving?

Make sure your subscription moves with you!

To notify us of your new address, find your **Clinics Account Number** (located on your mailing label above your name), and contact customer service at:

Email: journalscustomerservice-usa@elsevier.com

800-654-2452 (subscribers in the U.S. & Canada)
314-447-8871 (subscribers outside of the U.S. & Canada)

Fax number: 314-447-8029

**Elsevier Health Sciences Division
Subscription Customer Service
3251 Riverport Lane
Maryland Heights, MO 63043**

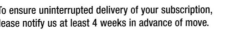

*To ensure uninterrupted delivery of your subscription, please notify us at least 4 weeks in advance of move.

ELSEVIER